The Evidence
for Urology

Edited by

Chris Dawson & Gordon Muir

Publisher

tfm Publishing Limited
Castle Hill Barns
Harley
Shrewsbury
SY5 6LX
UK

Tel: +44 (0)1952 510061
Fax: +44 (0)1952 510192
E-mail: nikki@tfmpublishing.com
Web site: www.tfmpublishing.com

Design and layout: Nikki Bramhill
Cartoon on front cover: Barry Foley

First Edition   © 2005

ISBN 1 903378 19 2

Printed by Gutenberg Press Ltd., Gudja Road, Tarxien, PLA 19, Malta.

Tel: +356 21897037; Fax: +356 21800069.

Contents

Contributors

Jim M Adshead MD MA FRCS (Urol), Specialist Registrar, Urology, Queen Elizabeth Hospital, Birmingham, UK

Peter Alken MD, Professor of Urology, University Hospital, Mannheim, Germany

Mamun Al-Rashid MB BS (Lon), Senior House Officer, Urology, Edith Cavell Hospital, Peterborough, UK

Nadim Ayoub MD, Fellow in Laparoscopic Urology, Saint-Augustin Clinic, Bordeaux, France

Omer Baldo MB BS MRCS (Glas), Clinical Research Fellow, Urology, St James' University Hospital, Leeds, UK

G Richard D Batstone MA MB BChir MD FRCS (Urol), Consultant Urologist, Redcliffe Hospital, Queensland, Australia

Jeetesh Bhardwa MB ChB MRCS (Eng), Research Fellow, Urology, Barts and The London, Queen Mary's School of Medicine and Dentistry, University of London, London, UK

Alison Birtle MRCP FRCR, Senior Specialist Registrar, Clinical Oncology, The Royal Marsden Hospital, Sutton, Surrey, UK

Tatjana Bubanj MD, Registrar, Paediatric Urology, Debrousse Hospital, Lyon, France

Emanuele Caldarera MD, Consultant Urologist, Vincenzo Cervello Hospital, Palermo, Italy

Linda Cardozo MD FRCOG, Professor of Urogynaecology, King's College Hospital, London, UK

Srinath Chandrasekera MS FRCS FEBU, Senior Research Fellow, Urology, King's College Hospital, London, UK

Alaa Cheikhelard MD, Clinical Fellow, Paediatric Urology, Debrousse Hospital, Lyon, France

Kerry A Cheong BMBS FRACP, Clinical Research Fellow, Medical Oncology, Guy's Hospital, London, UK

Kathryn F Chrystal MB ChB FRACP, Clinical Research Fellow, Medical Oncology, Guy's Hospital, London, UK

Chris Dawson BSc MS FRCS, Consultant Urologist, Edith Cavell Hospital, Peterborough, UK

Salvatore De Marco MD, Senior Physician, Medical Oncology, San Camillo Forlanini Hospital, Rome, Italy

Delphine Demède MD, Resident, Paediatric Urology, Debrousse Hospital, Lyon, France

Cosimo De Nunzio MD, Consultant Urologist, Sant' Andrea Hospital, Rome, Italy

Mihir M Desai MD, Staff, Laparoscopic & Robotic Surgery, Glickman Urological Institute - Section of Laparoscopic and Robotic Surgery, The Cleveland Clinic Foundation, Cleveland, Ohio, USA

Alan P Doherty BSc MD FRCS (Urol), Consultant Urologist, Queen Elizabeth Hospital, Birmingham, UK

Ian Eardley MA MChir FRCS (Urol) FEBU, Consultant Urologist, St James' University Hospital, Leeds, UK

Michaela Feist-Schwenk MD, Registar, Urology, SLK Kliniken Heilbronn, Teaching Hospital, University of Heidelberg, Germany

Murray S Feldstein MD, Instructor of Urology, Mayo Clinic Scottsdale, Scottsdale, Arizona, USA

Mark R Feneley MD FRCS (Eng) FRCS (Urol), Senior Lecturer in Urological Oncology, Institute of Urology and Nephrology, University College London, London, UK

Richard S Foster MD, Professor of Urology, Indiana University Medical Center, Indianapolis, USA

Chris Fowler BSc MA MS FRCS (Urol) FEBU, Professor of Surgical Education, Honorary Consultant Urologist, Barts and The London, Queen Mary's School of Medicine and Dentistry, University of London, London, UK

Bruno Frea MD, Consultant Urologist and Professor of Urology, Urology Clinic, Department of Medical Sciences, University of Piemonte Orientale, Novara, Italy

Thomas Frede MD, Consultant Urologist, SLK Kliniken Heilbronn, Teaching Hospital, University of Heidelberg, Germany

Thomas Gelas MD, Registrar, Paediatric Surgery, Debrousse Hospital, Lyon, France

Elmar W Gerharz MD PhD, Reader in Urology, Julius Maximilians University Medical School, Würzburg, Germany

Inderbir S Gill MD MCh, Head of Laparoscopic & Robotic Surgery, Glickman Urological Institute - Section of Laparoscopic and Robotic Surgery, The Cleveland Clinic Foundation, Cleveland, Ohio, USA

Dragan Golijanin MD, Resident, Urology, University of Rochester School of Medicine, Rochester, New York, USA

Fernando Gómez Sancha MD, Consultant Urologist, Instituto de Cirugía Urológica Avanzada, Madrid, Spain

Paolo Gontero MD, Senior Lecturer and Consultant Urologist, Urology Clinic, Department of Medical Sciences, University of Piemonte Orientale, Novara, Italy

Stephen J Griffin MMedSc FRCS Ed, Specialist Registrar, Urology, Edith Cavell Hospital, Peterborough, UK

Bertrand Guillonneau MD, Professor of Urology, Memorial Sloan-Kettering Cancer Center, New York, USA

Paul Hadway MB BS MRCS (Eng), Research Fellow, Urology, St George's Hospital, London, UK

Peter G Harper LRCP MRCS MB BS MRCP, Consultant Medical Oncologist, Guy's Hospital, London, UK

Sarah J Harris MB BS MRCP FRCR, Consultant Clinical Oncologist, St Thomas' Hospital, London, UK

Mikael Hoch MD, Resident, Paediatric Urology, Debrousse Hospital, Lyon, France

Jean-Luc Hoepffner MD, Specialist in Laparoscopic Urology, Saint-Augustin Clinic, Bordeaux, France

Mette Holm MD, Specialist Registrar, Urology, Department of Growth and Reproduction, Rigshospitalet, Copenhagen, Denmark

Sonja Hunt BA MA PhD, Honorary Senior Research Fellow, Department of Public Health Sciences, University of Edinburgh, Edinburgh, Scotland

Adrian D Joyce MS FRCS (Urol), Consultant Urologist, St. James' University Hospital, Leeds, UK

Jihad H Kaouk MD, Staff, Laparoscopic & Robotic Surgery, Glickman Urological Institute - Section of Laparoscopic and Robotic Surgery, The Cleveland Clinic Foundation, Cleveland, Ohio, USA

Roger Kirby MD FRCS (Urol) FEBU, Professor of Urology, St George's Hospital, London, UK

Thomas Knoll MD, Assistant Professor of Urology, University Hospital, Mannheim, Germany

Donald L Lamm MD, Professor of Urology, Mayo Clinic Scottsdale, Scottsdale, Arizona, USA

Robert Lee MD, Professor and Vice-Chairman, Department of Radiation Oncology, Wake Forest University, School of Medicine, Winston-Salem, NC, USA

Lewis C Liew MB ChB FRCS (Ed) FAMS (Urol), Consultant Urologist, National University Hospital, Singapore

Ralph Madeb MD, Resident, Urology, University of Rochester School of Medicine, Rochester, New York, USA

Asa Månsson RN PhD, Lecturer, University of Lund, Sweden

Wiking Månsson MD PhD, Associate Professor of Urology, University Hospital, Lund, Sweden

Edward M Messing MD, WW Scott Professor of Urology, University of Rochester School of Medicine, Rochester, New York, USA

Jon-Paul Meyer MRCS, Specialist Registrar in Urology, Royal Berkshire Hospital, Reading, UK

Pierre Mouriquand MD FRCS (Eng), Professor of Paediatric Urology, Debrousse Hospital, Lyon, France

Gordon Muir FRCS (Urol) FEBU, Consultant Urological Surgeon, King's College Hospital, London, UK

Chris Parker BA MRCP MD FRCR, Senior Lecturer in Clinical Oncology, Institute of Cancer Research & The Royal Marsden Hospital, Sutton, Surrey, UK

Matthew Parsons MB ChB MRCOG, Clinical and Research Fellow, Urogynaecology, King's College Hospital, London, UK

Heather Payne MRCP FRCR, Consultant Clinical Oncologist, The Meyerstein Institute of Oncology, The Middlesex Hospital, London, UK

Johan Poulsen MD FEBU, Consultant Urologist, Aalborg University Hospital, Denmark and King's College Hospital, London, UK

Jens J Rassweiler MD, Professor of Urology, SLK Kliniken Heilbronn, Teaching Hospital, University of Heidelberg, Germany

Paul S Sidhu MRCP FRCR, Consultant Radiologist, King's College Hospital, London, UK

Rashmi Singh BSc FRCS, Specialist Registrar, Urology, St George's Hospital, London, UK

Massimiliano Spaliviero MD, Fellow, Laparoscopic & Robotic Surgery, Glickman Urological Institute - Section of Laparoscopic and Robotic Surgery, The Cleveland Clinic Foundation, Cleveland, Ohio, USA

Seshadri Sriprasad MSc (Urol) FRCS FRCS (Urol), Specialist Registrar, Urology, King's College Hospital, London, UK

Cora N Sternberg MD FACP, Chief Physician, Medical Oncology, San Camillo Forlanini Hospital, Rome, Italy

Svetozar Subotic MD, Registar, Urology, SLK Kliniken Heilbronn, Teaching Hospital, University of Heidelberg, Germany

Dogu Teber MD, Senior Registrar, Urology, SLK Kliniken Heilbronn, Teaching Hospital, University of Heidelberg, Germany

A Karim Touijer MD, Urologic Oncology Fellow, Memorial Sloan-Kettering Cancer Center, New York, USA

Alberto Trucchi MD FEBU, Assistant Professor of Urology, Sant' Andrea Hospital, Rome, Italy

Andrea Tubaro MD FEBU, Associate Professor of Urology, Sant' Andrea Hospital, Rome, Italy

Hein Van Poppel MD PhD FEBU, Chairman & Professor of Urology, University Hospital Gasthuisberg, Leuven, Belgium

Kilian Walsh MB MSc (Urol) FRCS (Urol), Consultant Urological Surgeon, King's College Hospital, London, UK

Nicholas A Watkin MA MChir FRCS (Urol), Consultant Urologist, St George's Hospital, London, UK

Hugh N Whitfield MA MChir FRCS FEBU, Consultant Urologist, Royal Berkshire Hospital, Reading, UK

Oliver Wiseman MA FRCS, Specialist Registrar, Urology, Edith Cavell Hospital, Peterborough, UK

Gang Zhu MD PhD, Consultant Urologist, Beijing Hospital, Beijing, China

The Editors

Chris Dawson BSc MS FRCS

Chris Dawson is a consultant urological surgeon working at The Edith Cavell Hospital, Peterborough, and The Fitzwilliam Hospital, Peterborough, where his interests are oncology in general and prostate cancer in particular. He qualified in Medicine from University College Hospital London in 1986. His post-fellowship urological training included time at The Battle Hospital in Reading, The Institute of Urology in London, and The Edith Cavell Hospital in Peterborough. Chris has worked as a consultant urologist in Peterborough for eight years and has been Lead Clinician for the department for the last three years. Chris has a wife and two children and keeps fit in his spare time by practising Aikido (in which he holds a first degree black belt) and running Marathons.

Gordon Muir FRCS (Urol) FEBU

Gordon Muir is a consultant urological surgeon working at King's College Hospital, and the Lister Hospital, London, where his interests are in minimally invasive treatment of prostate disease, andrology and the teaching and assessment of surgical practice. He qualified in medicine at the University of Glasgow and spent time in active service as an Army medical officer; his postgraduate training in surgery and urology took place in London at St George's and the Royal Marsden Hospitals as well as spells in France, Egypt and Italy. Gordon has a wife and two children. He relaxes with opera, poetry and malt whisky. Despite a relative lack of both fitness and cruciate ligaments he still tries to spend as much spare time as possible on skis.

Dedications

Gordon's dedication:
To my family

Chris's dedication:
To Rachel and James, who light up my life

Introduction

Using evidence-based medicine in urology

Chris Dawson BSc MS FRCS

Consultant Urologist

EDITH CAVELL HOSPITAL, PETERBOROUGH, UK

What is evidence-based medicine?

Evidence-based medicine (EBM) has been defined as the "conscientious, explicit and judicious use of current best evidence in making decisions about the care of individual patients" [1]. The practice arguably began in the 1970s with the work of Cochrane who was the first to suggest that healthcare decisions should be made on the basis of evidence of randomised controlled trials.

The term itself was first used in Canada in the 1980s to denote a learning strategy which embraced problem-based learning and research principles to inform diagnosis, treatment, and prognosis [2].

Where to find evidence-based medicine?

Despite the progress in EBM, for many urologists the process of gathering evidence remains a time-consuming task. Furthermore, recent reports suggest that EBM is not currently in widespread use within urology. One audit of four major urological journals revealed that only one third of publications conformed to high scientific criteria [3].

The development of the internet has revolutionised the way that all of us practise, and on-line information retrieval is the modern equivalent of a trip to the library in former years. Many sources of EBM are now available including the internet sites listed in Table 1.

Why should we use EBM?

One of the main reasons for supporting the use of EBM in medicine in general, and urology in particular, is the rate of change of new practices, and the increasing tendency for sub-specialisation in urology. Faced with both of these facts it is difficult, if not impossible, to keep pace with new developments. If one then considers the relative paucity of scientific criteria available in most current journals [3], the problem becomes even more significant. How do we know that what we are reading or researching contains the best current evidence without the knowledge that stringent EBM principles are adhered to?

Without a way of critically appraising all the evidence before them there is no way for the urologist to decide which information is worth incorporating into clinical practice.

How do we practice EBM?

EBM is best practised by following five sequential steps:

1. Formulating an answerable question from the available clinical evidence.
2. Finding the best evidence to answer that question.
3. Critically evaluating the evidence.
4. Integrating that appraisal into our clinical practice.
5. Assessing the effectiveness of the above steps.

Formulating the initial question

When formulating the initial question the "PICO" mnemonic is useful and frequently quoted by EBM sites:

P Patient or problem.
I Intervention.
C Comparison intervention.
O Outcomes.

Considering a relevant problem in urology a question might be phrased like this:

P In patients with renal cancer.
I Is regular follow-up.
C Better than no follow-up.
O When considering risk of recurrence?

Only by structuring a question in this fashion is it possible to decide which evidence to accept or reject.

Finding the evidence

Some useful internet sources are quoted below in Table 1. As well as providing information about the nature and use of EBM, these sites also provide access to on-line databases and information resources.

Evaluating the evidence

The evidence present from both on-line and journal sources will be of varying quality and content. Fortunately, the practice of EBM has established some guidelines. The levels of evidence and grades of evidence used in this book are shown in Tables 2 and 3 and are widely used in EBM material.

Integrating the evidence into clinical practice

Having established the current evidence base for an individual's clinical practice, the next step is to amend that practice in line with the new evidence. There are many similarities in this regard to the use of audit which is now in widespread use in medicine. In some cases this may lead to a completely new way of working based on the new evidence, and in others the comfort of knowing that one's clinical practice is state-of-the-(evidence)-art!

Table 1. Sources of EBM information.

Centre for evidence-based medicine	http://www.cebm.net/index.asp
EBM on-line (subscription service)	http://ebm.bmjjournals.com/
Centre for evidence-based medicine	http://www.cebm.utoronto.ca/
Bandolier	http://www.jr2.ox.ac.uk/bandolier/
EBM Toolkit	http://www.med.ualberta.ca/ebm/ebmintro.htm
Evidence-based medicine (University of Massachusetts)	http://library.umassmed.edu/EBM/
Healthweb	http://healthweb.org/browse.cfm?subjectid=39
Netting the evidence	http://www.shef.ac.uk/scharr/ir/netting/
LHS Peoria, Illinois	http://www.uic.edu/depts/lib/lhsp/resources/ebm.shtml
Centre for Health Evidence	http://www.cche.net/usersguides/main.asp

Table 2. Levels of evidence.

Level	Type of evidence
Ia	Evidence obtained from systematic review of meta-analysis of randomised controlled trials
Ib	Evidence obtained from at least one randomised controlled trial
IIa	Evidence obtained from at least one well-designed controlled study without randomisation
IIb	Evidence obtained from at least one other type of well-designed quasi-experimental study
III	Evidence obtained from well-designed non-experimental descriptive studies, such as comparative studies, correlation studies and case studies
IV	Evidence obtained from expert committee reports or opinions and/or clinical experience of respected authorities

Table 3. Grades of evidence.

Grade of evidence	Evidence
A	At least one randomised controlled trial as part of a body of literature of overall good quality and consistency addressing the specific recommendation (evidence levels Ia and Ib)
B	Well-conducted clinical studies but no randomised clinical trials on the topic of recommendation (evidence levels IIa, IIb, III)
C	Expert committee reports or opinions and/or clinical experience of respected authorities. This grading indicates that directly applicable clinical studies or good quality are absent (evidence level IV)

Assessing the effectiveness

After a period of new practice the final step in this feedback loop is to audit the change or practice to see what, if any, difference has been made to clinical care. At this point the loop may start again with the formulation of a new clinical question

What is the need for this book?

As stated above, the use of EBM is certainly increasing but is still not in widespread use in most urology departments. Information for clinicians is available from a wide number of sources but, faced with a busy clinical workload, keeping up-to-date with current literature remains a daunting task for most.

The *Evidence for Urology* has been written with busy urologists in mind. The 40 chapters contained in this book have been written by authors across the clinical spectrum with input from authors of world renown in many cases.

Put simply, this book has taken 40 relevant clinical questions in urology and surveyed the current evidence for these topics according to EBM principles. The authors were asked to quote levels and grades of evidence for each major point, and to provide a summary at the end of each chapter with the major points of interest.

The authors are to be congratulated for producing this unique work in evidence-based urology. From this point on we hope that the use of EBM in urology will grow stronger and that, in the future, urologists will become better informed through the use of EBM.

References

1. Sackett DL, *et al*. Evidence-based medicine. What it is and what it isn't. *BMJ* 1996; 312: 71-2.
2. Gillenwater JY, Gray M. Evidence: What is it, Where do we find it, and How do we use it? *Eur Urol* 2003; Supplements 2: 3-9.
3. Månsson W. Evidence-Based Urology - A Utopia? *Eur Urol* 2004; 46: 143-146.

Chapter 1

Circumcision: harmful or not?

Tatjana Bubanj MD
Registrar, Paediatric Urology
Thomas Gelas MD
Registrar, Paediatric Surgery
Pierre Mouriquand MD FRCS (Eng)
Professor of Paediatric Urology

DEBROUSSE HOSPITAL, LYON, FRANCE

Circumcision is one of the oldest surgical procedures performed on humans and continues to evoke passionate discussions between pro and anti circumcision groups. It is also one of the most common procedures performed either inside or outside hospitals. One author [1] has commented that "the surface of foreskin removed each year in Britain would cover a football pitch". Three thousand one hundred and thirty-six articles were found on the Medline data base with circumcision.

In this chapter, circumcisions on cultural grounds are not considered, and only circumcisions performed for medical reasons are evaluated.

Introduction: where do we stand today?

Medical indications for circumcision are rather limited since it is now commonly accepted that a tight foreskin is a physiological feature in boys under three years of age [2]. Only 3% of male newborns have a retractable foreskin and 90% become retractile by the age of three. The number of medical indications has decreased even more with less invasive treatments aiming at loosening up the prepuce, such as preputioplasty and local steroids. Local application of

betamethasone on the tight prepuce each day for six weeks leads to a retractable foreskin in 87% cases with no described side effects [3] **(IIb/B)**.

The current indications for circumcision are:-

- Recurrent foreskin infections (incidence reported at 4% by Escala [4]).
- Scarred foreskin due to balanitis xerotica obliterans (BXO) (incidence is under 1% according to Kizer [5]) **(III/B)**. This incidence is increased in blacks compared to whites.
- Recurrent urinary tract infections (UTI) in children with severe underlying urological anomalies.

Beside these common medical indications, some have suggested that circumcision reduces the risk of cancer of the penis, cervical cancer and sexually transmitted diseases.

Is circumcision harmful?

Circumcision could be considered a dangerous procedure when one considers the multiple complications reported in the literature which vary from 2% to 10% of cases according to Williams and Kapila 1993 [6]. If per-, or post-circumcision blood loss, local infection and bad cosmetic results are the most commonly reported complications, the range of incidence of complications varies considerably from one report to another. For example, Ozdemir [7] reported a complication rate reaching 85% in circumcisions performed traditionally outside hospitals with much more favourable outcomes when the patients were circumcised in an operating room **(IIb/B)**. Conversely, Wiswell and Geschke [8] screening 136,086 boys in the US Army found 0.19% complications of circumcision **(III/B)** mainly represented by local infection, haemorrhage, and surgical trauma. The same group reports that the incidence of complications in the circumcised group approaches the incidence of UTI among uncircumcised male infants **(III/B)**.

One of the most frequently missed complications is meatal stenosis because most circumcised children do not have follow-up visits. This complication was not reported by Wiswell but was identified in 12 cases over a period of three years in the Department of Paediatric Surgery of Cambridge [9] **(IV/C)**. The cause of meatal stenosis following circumcision remains under discussion. It could be a non-physiological exposure of the mucosa of the urethral meatus rubbing on the underwear or nappies causing inflammation and subsequent stenosis. Alternatively, it could also be an ischaemic lesion of the meatus due to the fact that the frenular artery is commonly divided. This artery gives the blood supply to the glanular urethra and meatal mucosa.

Insufficient circumcision, persistent preputial adhesions, skin bridges, amputation of the glans, urethral fistula, skin retraction, granulomas, and concealed penis are also reported with very low levels of evidence (mostly case reports).

Pain and circumcision

Penile block anaesthesia is as good as caudal anaesthesia with fewer side effects [10] **(Ib/A)**. Local anaesthesia with EMLA cream is effective at reducing postoperative pain [11] **(Ib/A)**. The ring block anaesthesia is the most effective compared to EMLA cream or penile block anaesthesia [12] **(Ib/A)**.

Sexual consequences of circumcision

Although some report [13] that there is no difference in the male sexual lives before and after circumcision, these studies are all highly flawed as most males had a circumcision for medical reasons which obviously altered their sexual lives **(IIb/B)**. Furthermore, the follow-up of these men was short (12 weeks). These views seem to be shared in Masters and Johnson's study [14] **(IV/C)**, which also has major bias in the methodology.

Conversely, Taylor [15] suggested an histological basis to penile sensitivity in uncircumcised males **(IIb/B)**. Fink [16] reported mixed conclusions with no change in sexual activities between the two groups, and improved satisfaction in circumcised men, although 38% perceived some difficulty after this procedure **(III/B)**.

Female partners seem to prefer uncircumcised males [17], although here again there is huge bias in this study **(III/B)**. In both papers, the methodology used should be considered with caution as this kind of evaluation is highly subjective.

Circumcision: not harmful?

Does circumcision prevent UTI?

The foreskin is thought to be a natural reservoir of bacteria which could expose the male child to recurrent UTI. The infant prepuce has a natural flora (*E. Coli* and *Proteus*) and this seems to disappear when the foreskin becomes fully retractable.

The mucosal surface of the glans [18] may play an important role in the adhesion of some pathogenic bacteria **(IIb/B)**. Non-keratinized surfaces like the glans facilitate the adhesion of some bacteria such as P-fimbriated *E. Coli*, which are commonly involved in UTI. Wiswell [19] compared the bacterial population of the urethral meatus in two groups and noticed a significant increase in uncircumcised men **(IIb/B)**. In another study, Wiswell [20] screened 136,086 men in the US Army and noticed a significant difference in terms of UTI between the two groups, with the uncircumcised males being more prone to UTI than the circumcised ones (p<0.0001) **(III/B)**. These conclusions were also confirmed in a subsequent study run by Wiswell [21] with male infants for whom the risk of UTI was 12 times higher if they were not circumcised. Schoen [22] reached the same conclusions in a study following 14,893 male infants **(IIb/B)**. To [23] estimated the risk of UTI in the circumcised male infant population at 0.34 per 1000, compared to 1.54 per 1000 in the uncircumcised group **(IIb/B)**. However, the magnitude of the positive effect of circumcision seems to be much less than initially thought.

Does circumcision reduce the risk of penile cancer?

The incidence of penile cancer is so low (<1:100,000) that the benefit of circumcision is impossible to establish. Maden [24] reported a risk 3.2 times higher in the uncircumcised group, a result which must be questioned as many other factors may affect the incidence of this cancer such as smoking, genital warts, and number of sexual partners **(III/B)**. Another study from Brinton [25] reported an increase of 32.9 times in uncircumcised males with the same bias as the previous study.

Does circumcision reduce the risk of cervical cancer?

There is a well established relationship between cervical cancer and herpes virus infection (HPV) [26]. Circumcised males carry less HPV (5.5%) than uncircumcised males (19.6%) [27] **(IIb/B)**. However, there may be other ethnical factors which are important in the development of cervical cancers.

Does circumcision reduce the risk of HIV infection?

Moses [28] stated that the change of glans surface after circumcision may reduce the risk of HIV infection **(III/B)**. The foreskin can be traumatized during intercourse and might be an entry to viruses especially if other sexual diseases coexist. These conclusions were considered as overestimated by De Vincenzi [29] **(III/B)**. Van Howe [30] produced a meta-analysis and stated that circumcision does not prevent HIV infection and could even facilitate it **(III/B)**.

Reynolds [31] prospectively studied a population of Indian men attending sexually transmitted disease clinics and reported that circumcised men have a lower risk of HIV1 infection than uncircumcised men **(III/B)**. There is thus no consensus on this issue.

Conclusions

This procedure which is considered by some as a sexual mutilation, still raises incredibly passionate discussions as there is a very strong (and old) cultural and religious background. One should not ignore the commercial implications of circumcision which represents a substantial number of cases in some practices. Although current medical indications of removing the foreskin are rather limited, it seems that this procedure may help to reduce urinary tract infections especially in males with underlying urinary tract anomalies. Most indications of circumcision are based more on empirical medicine than on scientific evidence.

Chapter 1

Recommendations	Evidence level

Is circumcision associated with a significant number of complications?

- Yes, especially when performed outside the medical environment. — IIb/B
- The incidence of complications of circumcision approaches the incidence of UTI in uncircumcised males. — IIIb/B
- Late complications such as meatal stenosis are often ignored as these patients are rarely followed. — IV/C

Analgesia and circumcision

- Ring block anaesthesia is the most effective method. — Ib/A

Impact of circumcision on sexual life

- There are no statistically significant changes of sexual function in circumcised males. — IIb/B
- Women prefer vaginal intercourse with an anatomically complete penis. — III/B
- A very subjective issue which should be interpreted with great caution.

Does circumcision prevent UTI?

- The foreskin is a bacterial reservoir and uncircumcised infants have a 12-times higher risk of developing a UTI. — IIb/B
- Circumcision may reduce this risk but the magnitude of this effect is significantly less than previously estimated. — IIb/B

Does circumcision prevent penile cancer?

- The risk of penile cancer is 3.2 times greater in uncircumcised males. — III/B
- The numbers are so small that statistically valid studies do not exist.
- Other factors are certainly involved.

Does circumcision reduce the risk of cervical cancer?

- As circumcision reduces the risk of herpes virus infection, it is associated with a reduced risk of cervical cancer for the sexual partners although, here again, other factors are involved. — IIb/B

Does circumcision reduce the risk of HIV infection?

- There are contradictory publications. — III/B

Chapter 1

8

References

1. Rickwood AMK. The prepuce. *Essentials of Paediatric Urology* 2002: 181-188.
2. Gairdner D. The fate of foreskin. *BMJ* 1999; 2: 1433-1437.
3. Ashfield JE, Nickel KR, Siemens DR, MacNeily AE, Nickel JC. Treatment of phimosis with topical steroids in 149 children. *J Urol* 2003; 169(3): 1106-8.
4. Escala JM, Rickwood AMK. Balanitis. *Br J Urol* 1989; 63: 196-197.
5. Kizer WS, Prarie T, Morey AF. Balanitis xerotica obliterans: epidemiologic distribution in an equal access health care system. *South Med J* 2003; 96(1): 9-11.
6. Williams N, Kapila L. Complications of circumcision. *Br J Surg* 1993; 80: 1231-36.
7. Ozdemir E. Significantly increased complications risk with mass circumcision. *Br J Urol* 1997; 80: 136-9.
8. Wiswell TE, Geschke DW. Risk from circumcision during the first month of life compared with those for uncircumcised boys. *Pediatrics* 1989; 83: 1011-1015.
9. Persad R, Sharma S, McTavish J, Imber C , Mouriquand PDE. Clinical presentation and pathophysiology of meatal stenosis following circumcision. *Br J Urol* 1995; 75 (1): 91-3.
10. Gauntlett I. A comparison between local anaesthetic dorsal nerve block and caudal bupivacaine with ketamine for pediatric circumcision. *Paediatr Anaesth* 2003; 13(1): 38-42.
11. Choi WY, Irwin MG, Hui TW, Lim HH, Chan KL. EMLA cream versus dorsal penile nerve block for postcircumcision analgesia in children. *Anest Analg* 2003; 96(2): 369-9.
12. Lander J, Brady-Fryer B, Metcalfe JB, Nazarali S, Muttitt S. Comparison of ring block, dorsal penile nerve block, and topical anesthesia for neonatal circumcision: a randomized controlled trial. *JAMA* 1997; 278(24): 2157-62.
13. Collins S, Upshaw J, Rutchik S, Ohannessian C, Ortenberg J, Albertsen P. Effects of circumcision on male sexual function: debunking a myth? *J Urol* 2002; 167: 2111-2112.
14. Masters WH, Johnson VE. *Human Sexual Response*. Little Brown, Boston, 1966.
15. Taylor JR, Lockwood AP, Taylor AJ. The prepuce: specialized mucosa of the penis and its loss to circumcision. *Br J Urol* 1996; 77: 291-295.
16. Fink KS, Carson CC, DeVellis RF. Adult circumcision outcomes study: effect on erectile function, penile sensitivity, sexual activity and satisfaction. *J Urol* 2002; 167: 2113-2116.
17. O'Hara K, O'Hara J. The effect of male circumcision on the sexual enjoyment of the female partner. *BJU Int* 1999; 83: 79-84.
18. Fussell EN, Kaack MB, Cherry R, Roberts JA. Adherence of bacteria to human foreskins. *J Urol* 1988; 140(5): 997-1001.
19. Wiswell TE, Miller GM, Gelston HM Jr, *et al.* Effect of circumcision status on periurethral bacterial flora during the first year of life. *J Pediatr* 1988; 113: 442-446.
20. Wiswell TE, Geschke DW. Risk from circumcision during the first month of life compared with those for uncircumcised boys. *Pediatrics* 1989; 83: 1011-1015.
21. Wiswell TE. Prepuce presence portends prevalence of potentially perilous periurethral pathogens. *J Urol* 1992; 148: 739-742.
22. Schoen EJ, Colby CJ, Ray GT. Newborn circumcision decreases incidence and costs of urinary tract infections during the first year of life. *Pediatrics* 2000; 105: 789-793.
23. To T, Agha M, Dick PT, Feldman W. Cohort study on circumcision of newborn boys and subsequent risk of urinary-tract infection. *Lancet* 1998; 352: 1813-16.
24. Maden C, Sherman KJ, Beckmann AM, *et al.* History of circumcision, medical conditions and sexual activity and risk of penile cancer. *J Nat Cancer Inst* 1993; 85: 19-24.
25. Brinton LA, Jun-Yao L, Shou-De R, *et al.* Risk factors for penile cancer: results from a case-control study in China. *Int J Cancer* 1991; 47: 504-509.
26. Bosch FX, Manos MM, Munoz N, *et al.* Prevalence of human papillomavirus in cervical cancer: a worldwide perspective. *J Nat Cancer Inst* 1995; 87: 796-802.
27. Castellsague X, Bosch FX, Munoz N, Meijer CJ, Shah KV, de Sanjos Eluf-Neto J, Ngelangel CA, Chichareon S, Smith JS, Herrero R, Mor V, Franceschi S. International Agency for Research on Cancer Multicenter Cervical Study Group: male circumcision, penile human papilomavirus infection, a cervical cancer in female partners. *N Engl J Med* 2002; 346(15): 1105-12.
28. Moses S, Plummer FA, Bradley JE, *et al.* The association between lack of male circumcision and risk for HIV infection: a review of the epidemiological data. *Sex Transm Dis* 1994; 21: 201-210.
29. De Vincenzi I, Mertens T. Male circumcision: a role in HIV prevention? *AIDS* 1994; 8: 153-160.
30. Van Howe RS. Circumcision and HIV infection: review of the literature and meta-analysis. *Int J STD and AIDS* 1999; 10: 8-16.
31. Reynolds SJ, Shepard ME, Risbud AR, Gangakhedkar RR, Brookmeyer RS, Divekar AD, Mehendale SM, Bollinger RC. Male circumcision and risk of HIV-1 and other sexually transmitted infections in India. *Lancet* 2004; 363: 1039-1040.

Chapter 2

Penile preserving strategies for penile carcinoma

Paul Hadway MB BS MRCS (Eng)

Research Fellow, Urology

Nicholas Watkin MA MChir FRCS (Urol)

Consultant Urologist

ST GEORGE'S HOSPITAL, LONDON, UK

Introduction

Carcinoma of the penis is a rare disease. The incidence in England and Wales is 1.2-1.5 per 100,000 per year, very similar to that seen in other western countries [1]. In Africa, Asia and parts of South America, however, penile cancer accounts for up to 20% of all malignancies in men [2]. More than 95% of penile cancers are primary squamous cell carcinoma, the rest consisting of melanomas, sarcomas and basal cell carcinomas. Due to the rarity of the disease, and of particular relevance to this chapter, there is an absence of large randomised trials. Therefore, many guidelines on management remain controversial as they are based on small retrospective single institute series.

Historically, radical surgery and radiotherapy has been the mainstay of treatment. Surgical amputation undoubtedly provides excellent loco-regional oncological control. It is, however, associated with significant psychological morbidity as well as urinary and sexual dysfunction [3] **(III/B)**. For these reasons there has been a pressure to develop improved penile preserving therapies, with the aim of good oncological control with minimal anatomical and functional disruption. In the UK, where only 15% of tumours invade the corpora cavernosum at presentation, the vast majority will be amenable to such intervention. Early diagnosis is the key factor in selection of such treatments. Radical radiotherapy on the other hand is penile preserving, but it will often leave the patient with disfigurement and dysfunction. Salvage surgery will be required as a consequence in 20-40% of patients.

The purpose of this chapter is to review current ideas regarding various penile preserving strategies for penile cancer with the relevant evidence where available (Figure 1).

Diagnosis

The presentation of penile cancer is varied. The primary lesion can be an erythematous area, a nodular growth, ulceration or may present with phimosis. A groin mass may be the first symptom reported. The clinical difference between pre-malignant and benign lesions is subtle. Invasive disease, however, is generally straightforward to diagnose, but can be made more difficult by the consequences of previous

Chapter 2

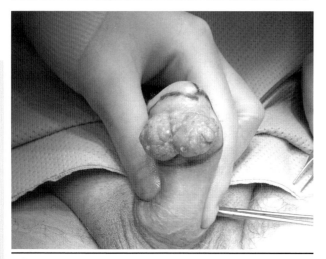

Figure 1. An exophytic penile squamous cell carcinoma.

radiotherapy. Furthermore, carcinoma *in situ* (CIS) and invasive disease co-exist in 25% of patients, and thus histological diagnosis is mandatory to determine grade and pathological characterisation. It should be noted that patients who have undergone previous radiotherapy are at risk of deep necrosis following such biopsies [4] **(III/B)**. The TNM staging system for penile carcinoma was revised by the UICC in 2002 (Table 1). Grading with Broder's system subdivides tumours into well, moderate and poorly differentiated tumours [5].

Penile preserving strategies

These can be broadly divided into surgical and non-surgical methods. Surgery can be further subdivided into glans preserving and glans removing procedures.

Table 1. TNM classification of penile carcinoma.

A. Primary tumour

Tx: Primary tumour can not be assessed
Tis: Carcinoma *in situ*
Ta: Non-invasive verrucous carcinoma
T1: Invades subepithelial connective tissues
T2: Invades corpus spongiosum/cavernosum
T3: Invades urethra or prostate
T4: Invades adjacent structures

B. Regional lymph nodes

Nx: Regional lymph nodes can not be assessed
N0: No regional lymph node metastasis
N1: Metastasis in single superficial inguinal lymph node
N2: Metastasis in multiple or bilateral superficial inguinal lymph nodes
N3: Metastasis in deep inguinal or pelvic node(s), unilateral or bilateral

C. Distant metastasis

Mx: Distant metastasis can not be assessed
M0: No distant metastasis
M1: Distant metastasis

The former includes circumcision, laser ablation and glans resurfacing with a skin graft. The latter includes glansectomy with reconstruction and distal corporectomy and reconstruction. Non-surgical techniques include radiotherapy, chemotherapy and immunotherapy.

Penile preserving surgery

It is evident that conventional surgery has significant psychosexual effects on patients. Radical surgery is clearly the treatment of choice for stage T4, high grade stage T3 and proximal stage T2 disease. The need for this, however, has been contested recently in less advanced cases and those with lower grade tumours.

Several series have been published challenging the need for the conventional 2cm resection margin. Agrawal and colleagues examined 62 partial and total penectomy specimens, looking for extension of the cancer into the proximal 2cm clearance margin [6] (III/B). Their work showed that of 52 grade 1 and 2 tumours, only seven had positive margins at 5mm from the tumour. Twenty-five percent of the grade 3 tumours had extended up to 10mm from the tumour. Hoffman's group looked at surgical specimens from 14 patients following conventional operations. The series included seven patients whose resection margins were less than or equal to 10mm. At 33 months follow-up none of the patients had developed a recurrence. Furthermore, long-term survival does not appear to be compromised by local recurrence, as most are surgically salvageable [7] (III/B).

Glans preserving surgery

Circumcision

Circumcision is by far the commonest operation in the surgical management of penile carcinoma. There are very few cases of penile carcinoma in circumcised men in the world literature. Circumcision is indicated for primary curative therapy in low stage preputial disease [8] (III/B). Adequate clearance margins must be achieved. If the lesion is more extensive the excision may be extended onto the shaft skin or coronal sulcus as necessary [9,10] (III/B). Circumcision is always recommended prior to radiotherapy, allowing for accurate targeting and tumour definition. It also aids surveillance for local recurrence (IV/C).

Recurrence rates of up to 30% have been reported following circumcision [4,11] (III/B). The majority of these will occur in the first two years following resection [12] (III/B). Close postoperative surveillance is therefore essential. Salvage surgery of these has a high success rate and does not appear to affect the disease-specific survival [9,13] (III/B). If carcinoma *in situ* is present at the resection margin this can be treated with topical 5-fluorouracil or Imiquimod cream, and closely observed.

Laser ablation

Laser treatment is well utilised in the treatment of penile carcinoma, carbon dioxide (CO_2) and Nd:YAG being the most commonly used types. The main difference between these is their penetration potential; CO_2 laser has a longer wavelength and does not penetrate human tissues as well as Nd:YAG. Therefore, it is essential to assess tumour depth before starting laser treatment. This can be either accomplished with a biopsy or with magnetic resonance or ultrasound imaging. A depth of 4-6mm can be achieved with the Nd:YAG laser.

The CO_2 laser vaporises and coagulates surface tissues while the Nd:YAG laser can penetrate to deeper tissues. This technique offers excellent cosmetic and functional results, and may be carried out in the outpatient setting.

Several studies have been reported in the world literature, which support the use of laser in penile carcinoma. In 1995, Windhal reported the treatment of 19 patients; 8 managed with CO_2 laser therapy alone and 11 with CO_2 and Nd:YAG laser treatment. They reported two recurrences (11%), which were salvageable with further laser treatment. Both patients were disease-free at 12 and 52 months. A study by Shirahana and colleagues in 1998 [14] (III/B) demonstrates the importance of case selection. They took patients with carcinomas less than 6mm thick, based on MRI and ultrasound scan assessments. Ten

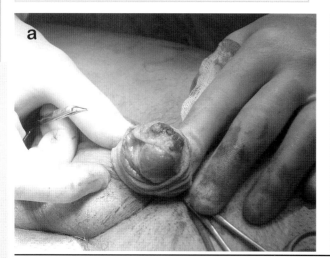
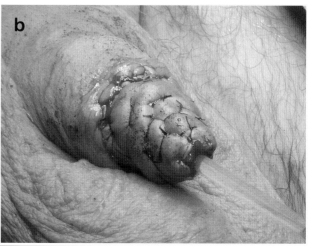

Figure 2. a) Glans resurfacing procedure for pre-invasive penile cancer. The epithelial and sub-epithelial tissues of half the glans have been dissected. b) Immediately post-glans resurfacing with split skin graft reconstruction.

cases of carcinoma *in situ* or stage T1 penile carcinoma were free of disease at six years. Two cases of stage T2 penile carcinoma were included in their series. These two patients were treated aggressively with a combination of chemoradiation and adjuvant laser therapy. Both were free of disease at seven and eight years of follow-up respectively. A few other studies demonstrate the potential advantage of aggressive combination therapies for advanced penile carcinomas [15,16] **(III/B)**.

The available data demonstrates that laser has significant cosmetic and functional advantages over conventional surgery. As with any organ-preserving therapy however, local recurrences are higher and close follow-up is essential to detect these early, and intervene without compromising patient survival. Patient selection is also very important. Late stage disease tends to be resistant to laser monotherapy. In such cases, combination therapy may be considered. Depth of invasion is also important, with tumours invading more than 6mm into tissue being unsuitable for laser surgery.

Glans resurfacing

This is a technique first described by Bracka for the treatment of severe balanitis xerotica obliterans

disease. The procedure has been adapted by the author for use in CIS and stage Ta/T1 disease. It involves removal of the glans epithelium and subepithelial tissues in quadrants. Frozen sections are then taken from the underlying corpus spongiosum, to confirm complete excision. The corpus spongiosus of the glans is then covered with a split thickness skin graft. As this is a new procedure, publication of the technique and follow-up data are awaited (Figure 2).

Glans removing surgery

Glansectomy and reconstruction

This is another new technique, involving the isolation and excision of the glans penis. It is indicated in tumours confined to the glans and prepuce. Frozen sections from the urethral stump and corporeal heads are recommended to ensure adequate excision. An end shaft urethrostomy is performed and a partial thickness skin graft applied to the corporal heads, to form a neoglans. A urethral catheter is left *in situ* for five days. Approximately 80% of all cases of invasive penile carcinoma are potentially amenable to this operation. To date the operation has not been widely reported. A series reported three cases of penile verrucous carcinoma, angiosarcoma and melanoma limited to the glans [17] **(III/B)**. All three underwent

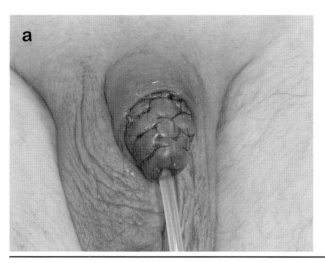
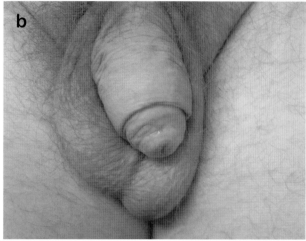

Figure 3. a) Immediately post-glansectomy with split skin graft reconstruction. b) Three months post-glansectomy with split skin graft reconstruction.

glansectomy with clear resection margins. No local recurrences were reported at follow-up of 12-48 months. Erections, sexual and urinary function was back to normal shortly after the operation in all cases. Hatzichristou and colleagues reported seven cases of verrucous carcinoma treated with glansectomy [18] **(III/B)**. In the series one patient required further surgery at three months for a local recurrence but all patients were alive and tumour-free at 18-65 months.

Watkin and Bracka, the surgeons accredited with the technique of glansectomy have two large series of patients. Watkin reported on 39 patients undergoing glansectomy, none of whom had developed local recurrence at 24 months follow-up [12]. Bracka has a similar sized group of patients, which is yet to be published. His results are similar in terms of outcome with over five years follow-up (personal communication). Early reports suggest this operation offers good cosmetic results, with preservation of urinary and sexual function (Figure 3).

Distal corporectomy and reconstruction

This more extensive technique is required if there is evidence of corporeal involvement, or if frozen sections of the corpora, urethra or tunica albuginea are positive. An extra 4cm can be gained by dividing the suspensory ligaments. A neoglans is then constructed from the corpora. The shaft skin is fully

mobilised to prevent later traction and shortening, and the denuded corporeal heads are then covered by a split thickness skin graft. The cosmetic outcome is better then for conventional surgery. Case selection is very important, as is close follow-up. The technique can also be used to salvage recurrences after radiotherapy or partial penectomy.

Non-surgical penile preserving strategies

Radiotherapy

This is a well established, first-line therapy for penile carcinoma [19] **(III/B)**. External beam radiotherapy (EBRT) or brachytherapy can be used. Brachytherapy can be divided into interstitial brachytherapy (IBRT) where the radiation source is implanted into the cancer, or plesiotherapy, where the radiation source surrounds the tumour.

EBRT is the most popular technique. The whole of the penis is irradiated, with the use of a wax mould to ensure an even distribution of radiation. A total dose of 50-70Gy is required, given in 15-30 daily sessions over 3-8 weeks on an outpatient basis. The obvious disadvantage is the duration of the regime and in addition, acute radiation reactions are common and often necessitate termination of treatment.

Chapter 2

IBRT involves implanting radioactive wires or needles, usually iridium-192, into the penis. The wires are held in place by two external templates, the distribution of holes along them ensuring an even administration of radiation. Again a dose of 50-70Gy is the aim. The duration of treatment is 5-7 days. Unfortunately, the treatment takes place in an isolation room, as an inpatient.

Plesiotherapy involves the placement of two moulds around the penis. The inner one straightens the penis and the outer is loaded with radioactive wires. Patient co-operation and dexterity are essential for successful treatment. The mould is applied for 12 hours a day, for a week. The patient is treated in isolation and a total dose of 60Gy is the target.

The biophysical advantage of brachytherapy, compared to EBRT, is the more targeted dose of radiation with fewer potential side effects. The patient has more control and treatment is shorter. The main disadvantage is the need for isolation.

The complication rates for all modes of radiotherapy are significant. Virtually all patients develop an acute radiation reaction (mucositis, skin irritation and tissue oedema). Late complications occur at varying rates, with up to 40% affected [20,21] (III/B). Urethral strictures occur in 15%-40% of patients [4, 22] (III/B). Skin changes such as telangiectasia, hypochromasia and superficial necrosis are common (Figure 4).

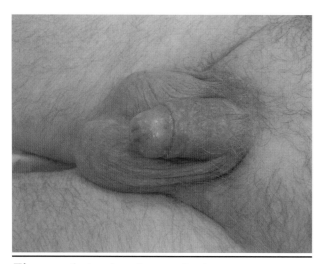

Figure 4. Penis after radiotherapy treatment. Marked telangiectasia present.

To date there are no prospective randomised trials assessing the effectiveness of radiotherapy compared with other treatments. Information from retrospective studies has been consistently reproducible [23,24] (III/B). Recurrence rates range from 15%-40%, which is higher than for conventional and penile preserving surgery. The mode of delivery of the radiotherapy does not appear to affect the outcome. As stated previously, the vast majority of the recurrences are surgically salvageable. The overall organ preservation rates are in the region of 60%-80%, with no compromise in five- and ten-year survival. However, functional and cosmetic impairment occur frequently.

Chemotherapy

Penile carcinomas are chemosensitive to a certain degree. Systemic chemotherapy has been used mainly in the palliative setting, for metastatic and advanced loco-regional disease [25-30] (III/B). It has also found a use in down-staging locally advanced tumours prior to surgery [4,31,32] (III/B). Only small series exist in the world literature. Bleomycin, cisplatin, methotrexate and vinblastine are the most frequently used agents, usually in combination with one another or with radiotherapy/immunotherapy [32,33] (III/B). Their response rate is often partial and short-lasting [30] (III/B). Recently, Cotsadze and co-workers [33] reported their experience in using systemic chemotherapy as a curative primary organ-preserving therapy for penile carcinoma. They treated 33 patients with four different chemotherapy regimes: bleomycin monotherapy (11 cases), vinblastine and bleomycin (11 cases), cisplatin and bleomycin (six cases) and cisplatin, vinblastine and bleomycin (six cases). They reported an overall 48.5% complete response rate after only one cycle of chemotherapy. Organ preservation was increased to 60.6% by adjuvant cryodestruction in partial responders. None of the stage T3 patients responded completely. The local recurrence rate was 18.7%, and all of these patients were salvaged surgically. The five- and ten-year survival rates were 78% and 73% respectively. There was no advantage in using multidrug chemotherapy compared to bleomycin monotherapy (III/B).

Mitropoulos and colleagues [32] (III/B) treated 12 cases (stage-T2/T3) with immunochemotherapy (cisplatin and interferon-α). They reported a 75% response rate. Four (33%) cases responded completely and five (42%) responded partially (defined as reduction in the size of tumour by more than 50%). They found a 50% local recurrence rate in the complete response group. All recurrences were surgically salvaged with amputation.

Immunotherapy

The reported use of immuno-monotherapy in penile carcinomas is limited to verrucous carcinomas (VC) [34] (III/B). Verrucous carcinomas are non-invasive (stage Ta) squamous cell carcinomas. They do not metastasize and have a good prognosis. Radiotherapy-induced anaplastic transformation of VC, however, has been reported [35] (III/B). There are only two reports of interferon-α monotherapy for VC both from the same institution [34] (III/B). The authors reported the successful use of subcutaneous interferon-α for three cases of VC in young individuals. They reported no significant systemic adverse reactions. One case was a patient with a recurrent tumour, who was refusing further surgery. He had five months of interferon treatment and was tumour-free at ten years follow-up. In the second case, interferon was used as a primary therapy in a patient, again, refusing surgery. He was treated for three months and he was tumour-free at seven years follow-up. Furthermore, a group from France reporting on the treatment of VC in other parts of the body, including a penile VC, concluded that interferon monotherapy can slow down the growth of tumours and can be used as an adjuvant therapy to surgical excision, but never prevents surgery or death [36] (III/B).

Conclusions

Definitive management of penile carcinomas is stage-dependent. There are no randomised prospective trials comparing treatment options. The vast majority of experts agree that stage Ta and T1, well/moderately differentiated carcinomas could be successfully treated with penile preserving therapies [37]. The management of stage T2 and low grade T3 tumours however, remains controversial. Careful case selection, based on both tumour and patient characteristics is required. NICE (National Institute for Clinical Excellence) has recently recommended that the management of these tumours should become more centralised and structured [38] (IV/C). This should allow teams to collaborate on important areas of management, which remain controversial.

Close follow-up is required after penile preserving therapies. Long-term recurrence rates are still unknown for many of these surgical techniques. From the small studies available it appears that local recurrence rates following radiotherapy, chemotherapy and immunotherapy are high. Functionally, patients undergoing penile preserving surgical procedures do better than those having conventional surgery, but these results should be critically compared to those undergoing radical radiotherapy. Finally, partial and radical penectomy should be reserved for the patient that presents with advanced disease.

Chapter 2

Chapter 2

Recommendations	Evidence level

- ◆ Conventional surgery is associated with psychological, sexual and urinary dysfunction. — III/B
- ◆ The need for a 2cm resection margin has been contested. — III/B
- ◆ The majority of local recurrences following surgery or radiotherapy will occur in the first two years. Therefore, close postoperative surveillance is essential. EAU guidelines for 2004 suggest two-monthly follow-up for the first two years, three-monthly for the third year and six-monthly thereafter [37]. — III/B
- ◆ Glans resurfacing and glansectomy are new techniques. Early results would suggest better cosmesis and function, when compared to conventional methods. Comparative studies will be required. — III/B
- ◆ Salvage surgery has a high success rate and survival rates appear unaffected by recurrences that are detected early. — III/B
- ◆ Radiotherapy is a well established treatment option, with various techniques available. It does have significant, early and late complication rates. A prospective randomised trial, comparing radiotherapy with other treatment modalities is required. — III/B
- ◆ Experience with immunotherapy is limited in penile cancer. It may play a role in those patients who refuse, or are too frail for surgery. Larger studies are required before conclusions can be drawn. — III/B

References

1. www.statistics.gov.uk. Cancer trends in England and Wales, 1950-1999.

2. Pow Sang MR, Benavente V, Pow Sang JE, *et al*. Cancer of the penis. *Cancer Control* 2002; 9: 305-314.

3. Opjordsmoen S, Fossa SD. Quality of life in patients treated for penile cancer. A follow-up study. *Br J Urol* 1994; 74(5): 652-657.

4. Pizzocaro G, Piva L, Tana S. Up-to-date management of carcinoma of the penis. *Eur Urol* 1997; 32: 5-15.

5. Broders AC. Squamous cell epithelioma of the skin. *Ann Surg* 1921; 73: 141.

6. Agrawal A, Pai D, *et al*. The histological extent of the local spread of carcinoma of the penis and its therapeutic implications. *BJU Int* 2000; 85(2): 299-301.

7. Hoffman M, Renshaw A, Loughlin KR. Squamous cell carcinoma of the penis and microscopic pathologic margins. How much margin is needed for local cure? *Cancer* 1999; 85(7): 1565-1568.

8. Bissada NK. Conservative extirpative treatment of cancer of the penis. *Urol Clin North Am* 1992; 19(2): 283-292.

9. McDougall WS, Kirchner FK, Edward RH, Killian LT. Treatment of carcinoma of the penis: the case of primary lymphadenectomy. *J Urol* 1986; 136: 38-41.

10. Das S. Penile amputation for the management of primary carcinoma of the penis. *Urol Clin North Am* 1992; 19(2): 277-282.

11. Colberg JW, Andriloe GL, *et al*. Surgical management of penile cancer. In: *Comprehensive Textbook of Genitourinary Oncology*. Vogelzang NJ, Scardino PT, Shipley WU, *et al*, Eds. Williams and Wilkins, Baltimore, 1999: 1103-1109.

12. Pietrzak P, Corbishley C, Watkin NA. Organ-sparing surgery for invasive penile cancer. Early follow-up data. *BJU Int* 2004; in press.

13. Lindegaard JC, Nielsen OS, *et al*. A retrospective analysis of 82 cases of cancer of the penis. *Br J Urol* 1996; 77(6): 883-890.

14. Shirahama T, Takemoto M, Nishiyama K, *et al*. A new treatment for penile conservation in penile carcinoma: a preliminary study of combined laser hyperthermia, radiation and chemotherapy. *Br J Urol* 1998; 82: 687-693.

15. Kuroda M, Tsushima T, Nasu Y. Hyperthermotherapy added to the multidisciplinary therapy for penile cancer. *Acta Med Okayama* 1993; 47: 169-174.

16. Obama T, Mitsuhata N, Yoshimoto J, Matsumura Y, Ohmori H. Combination therapy with continuous infusion of peplomycin, radiation and hyperthermia in advanced penile cancer: a case report. *Nishinihon J Urol* 1981; 43: 769-774.

17. Davis JW, Schellhammer PF, Schlossberg SM. Conservative surgical therapy for penile and urethral carcinoma. *Urology* 1999; 53: 386-392.

18. Hatzichristou DG, Apostolidis A, Tzortzis V, *et al.* Glansectomy: an alternative surgical treatment for Buschke-Lowenstein tumours of the penis. *Urology* 2001; 57: 966-9.

19. Srinivas V, Morse M, *et al.* Penile cancer: relation of node metastasis to survival. *J Urol* 1987; 137(5): 880-2.

20. Koch MO, Smith JA Jr. Local recurrence of squamous cell carcinoma of the penis. *Urol Clin North Am* 1994; 21(4): 739-743.

21. Gerbaulet A, Lambin P. Radiation therapy of cancer of the penis. Indications, advantages and pitfalls. *Urol Clin North Am* 1992; 19(2): 325-332.

22. Ravi R, Chaturvedi HK, Sastry DVLN. Role of radiation therapy in the treatment of carcinoma of the penis. *Br J Urol* 1994; 74: 646-651.

23. McLean M, Ahmed M, Warde P, *et al.* The results of primary radiation therapy in the management of squamous cell carcinoma of the penis. *Int J Radiat Oncol Biol Phys* 1993; 25(4): 623-8.

24. Horenblas S, van Tinteren H, *et al.* Squamous cell carcinomas of the penis. II. Treatment of the primary tumour. *J Urol* 1992; 147: 1533-1538.

25. Shammas FV, Ous S, Fossa SD. Cisplatin and 5-fluorouracil in advanced cancer of the penis. *J Urol* 1992; 147(3): 630-2.

26. Corral DA, Sella A, Pettaway CA, *et al.* Combination chemotherapy for metastatic or locally advanced genitourinary squamous cell carcinoma: a phase II study of methotraxate, cisplatin and bleomycin. *J Urol* 1998; 160(5): 1770-4.

27. Haas GP, Blumenstein BA, Gangliano RG, *et al.* Cisplatin, methotraxate and bleomycin for the treatment of carcinoma of the penis: a Southwest Oncology Group study. *J Urol* 1999; 161(6): 1823-5.

28. Roth AD, Berney CR, Rohner AS, *et al.* Intra-arterial chemotherapy in locally advanced or recurrent carcinomas of the penis and anal canal: an active treatment modality with curative potential. *Br J Cancer* 2000; 83(12): 1637-1642.

29. Kattan J, Culine S, Droz JP, *et al.* Penile cancer chemotherapy: twelve years' experience at Institut Gustave-Roussy. *Urology* 1993; 42(5): 559-562.

30. Ahmed T, Sklaroff R, Yagoda A. Sequential trials of methotrexate, cisplatin and bleomycin for penile cancer. *J Urol* 1984; 132(3): 465-8.

31. Bandieramonte G, Lepera P, Mogha D, Faustini M, Pizzocaro G. Neoadjuvant chemotherapy and conservative surgery for exophytic T1N0 carcinoma of the penis. Fourth International Congress on Anticancer Chemotherapy, Paris 1993, abstr 178.

32. Mitropoulos D, Dimopoulos MA, Kiroudi-Voulgari A, *et al.* Neoadjuvant cisplatin and interferon-alpha 2B in the treatment and organ preservation of penile carcinomas. *J Urol* 1994; 152(4): 1124-6.

33. Cotsadze D, Matveev B, Zak B, Mamaladze V. Is conservative organ-sparing treatment of penile carcinoma justified? *Eur Urol* 2000; 38: 306-312.

34. Maiche AG, Pyrhonen S. Verrucous carcinoma of the penis: three cases treated with interferon-alpha. *Br J Urol* 1997; 79: 481-3.

35. Fukunaga M, Yokoi K, Miyazawa Y, Hrada T, Ushigome S. Penile verrucous carcinoma with anaplastic transformation following radiotherapy. A case report with human papilloma virus typing and flow cytometric DNA studies. *Am J Surg Pathol* 1994; 18(5): 501-5.

36. Risse L, Negrier P, Dang PM, *et al.* Treatment of verrucous carcinoma with recombinant alfa-interferon. *Dermatology* 1995; 190(2): 142-4.

37. EAU guidelines on Penile Cancer. *Eur Urol* 2004; 46(1): 1-8.

38. National Institute for Clinical Excellence. Guidance on cancer services - Improving Outcomes in Urological Cancers - The Manual 2002: 83-85.

Chapter 2

Chapter 3

Management of lymph nodes in penile carcinoma

Rashmi Singh BSc FRCS
Specialist Registrar, Urology
Nicholas A Watkin MA MChir FRCS (Urol)
Consultant Urologist

ST GEORGE'S HOSPITAL, LONDON, UK

Introduction

In the western world, penile cancer is an uncommon malignancy. The number of new cases per year in the male population is only 1.2-1.5 per 100,000 [1]. This low incidence of penile cancer together with a lack of worldwide prospective randomised clinical trials has led to wide variation in treatment strategies. Although the management of this cancer is slowly evolving, certain aspects of treatment, particularly with regards to nodal disease, remain controversial and will be addressed in this chapter.

Anatomy of lymphatic drainage

Primary lymphatic drainage of squamous carcinoma of the penis is to the inguinal lymph node group and then secondarily to the iliac group. Metastatic disease appears to occur in an orderly stepwise fashion with regional lymphadenopathy pre-dating distant metastases.

The inguinal nodes can be divided into a large superficial group, which lie deep to the subcutaneous fat but above fascia lata and the smaller group lying around the fossa ovalis and deep to fascia lata. The deeper nodes receive afferent lymphatics from the superficial group and link up with the iliac nodes. The largest node in the deep group, known as Cloquet's node, lies beneath the inguinal ligament medial to the femoral vein. Anatomically, the inguinal node group can be divided into four sub-sections by drawing intersecting lines which pass through the sapheno-femoral junction. Metastases from penile cancer predominantly involve the nodes lying in the supero-medial quadrant.

The iliac or pelvic nodes are those situated around the iliac vessels and in the obturator fossa. Interestingly, although inguinal drainage from the penis appears to be bilateral, pelvic crossover does not appear to occur.

Prognostic importance of inguinal lymph node status

It is now well recognised that the most important prognostic factor for long-term survival in penile cancer is inguinal lymph node status. Data from a

Chapter 3

number of surgical series **(III/B)** suggest that approximately 50% (range 20%-96%) of patients have palpable inguinal lymph nodes at diagnosis of which up to 50% are due to tumour involvement, the remainder being enlarged due to inflammation/infection of the primary penile lesion. In those with pathological involvement of the nodes, average five-year survival rates of 60% (range 0%-86%) have been reported by the same series, depending on the number and extent of nodal metastases. In patients with non-palpable nodes, however, only 20% have been reported to have micrometastases [2,3] **(III/B)**. Inguinal lymphadenectomy in patients with small volume positive nodes is potentially curative, with a reported five-year survival of up to 80% [2,4] **(III/B)**. Multiple (greater than two), or bilateral node involvement and extracapsular tumour are adverse prognostic features. The prognostic implications of nodal status necessitate accurate assessment and surveillance of the inguinal regions in all patients with penile cancer.

Management of the patient with palpable lymph nodes

In those patients with palpable groin nodes at presentation, evidence suggests a beneficial role for routine inguinal lymphadenectomy. As mentioned previously, up to 50% of this group will subsequently be found to have positive nodes at pathological examination. The traditional approach of prolonged courses of antibiotics is less commonly practised now with a move towards early lymph node dissection in this group of patients. Whether bilateral lymphadenectomy should be performed in patients with only unilaterally palpable nodes remains controversial. Although bilateral dissections is the ideal in view of the fact that lymphatic drainage of the penis is bilateral, European guidelines [5] **(IV/C)** suggest a role for modified lymphadenectomy and frozen section initially on the contralateral side, with extension to full block dissection if tumour involvement is confirmed. In their series of over 200 cases, Ekstrom et al [6] observed that 50% of such patients were subsequently found to have positive nodes on the contralateral clinically "negative" side **(III/B)**.

In those patients presenting late with palpable lymph nodes whilst on surveillance, bilateral inguinal lymphadenectomy is an option. However, in those with a long disease-free interval and unilaterally palpable nodes only, dissection of the clinically positive side can be performed initially with close surveillance of the contralateral groin. The probability of developing late involvement of the contralateral groin nodes in this situation is around 10% [6] **(III/B)**.

Management of the patient with impalpable lymph nodes

One of the main dilemmas in the treatment of penile cancer lies with the group who are clinically node-negative at the time of presentation of the primary tumour. Should inguinal lymphadenectomy be performed as an adjunctive or prophylactic procedure in these patients of whom only 20% will be found to have histologically positive nodes [2,3]? **(III/B)**.

Routine prophylactic inguinal lymphadenectomy, although potentially curative, would "overtreat" 80% of cases and subject them to the significant complications associated with this operation (see below). The alternative option in patients who are clinically node negative is close surveillance with delayed lymphadenectomy as necessary, but this option carries the risk of missing occult metastases, present in around 20% of cases. The overall evidence from a number of studies suggests an improvement in survival in patients offered early versus late lymphadenectomy with only limited success of salvage procedures once metastases have developed [7-11] **(III/B)**. However, the results from many of these non-randomised studies are confounded by the small numbers of patients in the series and variability in the timing of the lymphadenectomy. Stratification of patients into risk groups based on histological features of the primary tumour has enabled management strategies to be developed for what remains a very controversial aspect of penile cancer. Currently, lymphadenectomy is recommended in those patients at high risk (greater than 50%) of nodal disease, i.e those with G3 or >T2 disease, those with G2T1 disease with adverse histological features eg. lymphovascular invasion or those not suitable for surveillance. The remaining intermediate and low risk patients i.e those with Tis (carcinoma *in situ*),

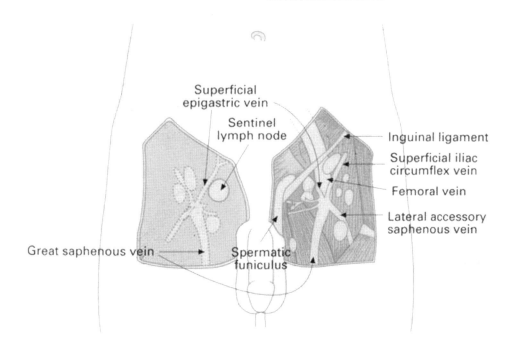

Figure 1. The superficial lymphatics can be anatomically described in quadrants. The sentinel node is in the superomedial group.

verrucous carcinoma (Ta) or G1/G2 T1 tumours have a less than 10% incidence of nodal involvement making them suitable candidates for surveillance [5] **(IV/C)**.

Surveillance of the inguinal regions

Those patients who have been selected for expectant management of the inguinal nodes require close surveillance. Patients should undergo clinical palpation of the nodes at 3-6 monthly intervals depending on risk. Physical examination alone may be inaccurate, with a sensitivity of 82% and a specificity of 79%, depending on the body habitus of the patient and whether there has been previous inguinal surgery [12] **(III/B)**. Radiological studies can be used as an adjunct but modalities such as CT and MRI have limitations in terms of their accuracy, particularly for the detection of lymph nodes at an early stage. Lymphangiography has now fallen out of favour in view of the technical difficulties associated with the procedure. Ultrasound (USS) is superior to CT for defining architectural changes suggestive of metastatic involvement in patients with impalpable

nodes. In combination with fine needle aspiration (FNA), the sensitivity and specificity of USS increases significantly and is currently the optimal investigation in patients who are clinically node-negative but at high risk of occult metastases. The technique can also be applied successfully in patients with palpable nodes in whom clinical examination has a specificity of only 50%. FNA in such cases has a false negative rate of only 15% [12-14] **(III/B)**.

Other non-invasive functional imaging techniques such as PET may become more important in the future but at present there are only limited data available.

Dynamic sentinel node biopsy

The relative unreliability of current clinical methods to detect occult lymph node metastases has provoked much interest in the application of sentinel lymph node mapping in penile cancer. The sentinel lymph node (SLN) is defined as the first node in the lymphatic group into which a primary tumour drains (Figure 1). The main afferent lymphatic from the tumour first drains into the SLN and therefore its tumour status

Chapter 3

accurately reflects the rest of the group. In other words, if the SLN is negative for metastases, the remainder of the lymph node group should also be negative. Conversely, if the SLN is positive, there is a strong likelihood that the other higher nodes in the group will also be involved. Lymphatic mapping and sentinel lymph node biopsy was first reported in 1977 by Cabanas in penile cancer and since then has been successfully applied to melanoma and breast cancer [15]. SLN mapping involves a pre-operative injection around the tumour with either intradermal isosulfan blue dye or Tc [99m] colloid sulphur in combination with a hand-held gamma probe, to localise the node. The advantages of the technique include the ability to provide the pathologist a limited number of lymph nodes for focused analysis and decreased morbidity. In penile cancer, the technique is a particularly valuable staging tool in the clinically node negative patient group. It enables the identification of those patients with early occult metastases who should proceed to a formal lymphadenectomy. The main disadvantages are the problems associated with

accurate identification of the true SLN and subsequent false negative rates. However, Horenblas et al reported a sensitivity of 80% for the detection of occult lymph node metastases using dynamic sentinel node biopsy [16] **(III/B)**. Akduman et al reported 100% accuracy of the technique in a small number of patients with intermediate risk penile cancer and impalpable groin nodes [17] **(III/B)**. In terms of survival, Lont et al propose that early detection of lymph node metastases using sentinel node biopsy and subsequent resection in clinically node negative T2-T3 penile cancer improves disease-specific three-year survival compared with surveillance (91% versus 79%, p=0.04) [18] **(IIb/B)**.

Dynamic sentinel lymph node biopsy is a promising and reliable technique for the detection of early lymph node metastases. Current recommendations are that SLN biopsy should not be used in patients with clinically positive nodes and should be reserved as an investigational technique in those with no obvious nodal involvement in whom the morbidity of unnecessary lymphadenectomy can be spared. Due to false negative results, close follow-up for the first two years following the procedure is essential so that prompt surgical intervention can be undertaken if necessary [5,14] **(IV/C)**.

Surgical techniques for inguinal lymphadenectomy

Inguinal lymphadenectomy can involve either dissection of the nodes superficial to fascia lata only or a complete block dissection with clearance of nodes deep to this layer and within the femoral triangle. This classical "radical" inguinal lymphadenectomy is associated with a complication rate of nearly 85% [9-11] **(III/B)**. Problems include lymphoedema, lymphocoele, deep vein thrombosis, wound infection and skin flap necrosis. As a result of these significant sequelae, a "modified" block dissection technique has been developed in an attempt to minimise morbidity without compromising tumour clearance [19-21] (Figure 2). This allows thick skin flaps with reduced external and inferior boundaries, preservation of the saphenous vein and no mobilisation of sartorius which maintains coverage of the femoral vessels.

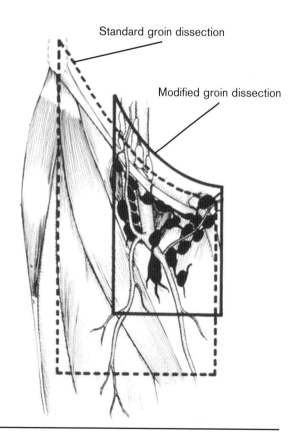

Standard groin dissection

Modified groin dissection

Figure 2. Boundaries of modified lymph node dissection are shown.

Both the superficial and modified lymph-adenectomy techniques are suitable staging tools for identifying micrometastases in patients with impalpable nodes and potentially avoid the need for radical block dissection.

Radiotherapy and the inguinal nodes

Radiotherapy is an alternative modality to surgical lymphadenectomy for the inguinal regions. Although there are no data from randomised controlled trials, the five-year survival rates in patients with inguinal metastases treated with surgery are far superior to those treated with radiotherapy (50% versus 25%) [22] **(IIb/B)**. In patients who are clinically node negative, there has been no demonstrable benefit of prophylactic groin radiotherapy in reducing the risk of late inguinal metastases [6,23] **(III/B)**. Moreover, radiotherapy also has significant morbidity associated with it. The inguinal regions tend to develop problems with maceration and ulceration and post-radiotherapy groins can be very difficult to follow-up with clinical examination. Currently, the recommended role for radiotherapy is in the palliative setting in those patients with bulky or fixed inoperable nodes (Figure 3), or as an adjuvant treatment after surgery in those patients with more than three positive nodes or extracapsular involvement, factors associated with a poor prognosis [2,4] **(III/B)**.

Management of the iliac nodes

The other controversial issue to address is the management of iliac nodes in patients with positive inguinal nodes. Despite the potentially curative role of inguinal node dissection, a proportion of these patients will have occult metastases in the iliac nodes or at distant sites. Patients with two or more positive inguinal nodes or extracapsular invasion have a 20%-30% risk of pelvic nodal involvement [7,13] **(IIa-III/B)** and could be considered for pelvic lymphadenectomy. Although surgery alone is unlikely to be curative once there is macroscopic disease within the pelvic nodes, five-year survival rates of up to 50% have been reported in cases with microscopic invasion [24,25] **(III/B)**. However, these studies contained very small numbers of cases and the average five-year survival

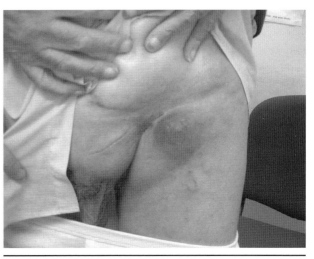

Figure 3. Large fixed inguinal nodes in an elderly patient are shown. These can potentially ulcerate.

for patients with positive pelvic nodes is around 10%. However, the procedure has the potential to improve loco-regional control and allows identification of those patients who may benefit from adjuvant therapy. In the absence of evidence from randomised controlled trials and only limited data from phase II studies, the optimal treatment and its timing remains controversial. Currently, the value of adjuvant pelvic radiotherapy or chemotherapy remains uncertain and such treatments should therefore be conducted within the context of controlled clinical trials. However, the precedent in other ano-genital squamous cell carcinomas (eg. vulva, anus and cervix) suggests that such lesions are likely to be radiosensitive and also that synchronous chemo-radiotherapy may be beneficial [26,27] **(Ib/A)**. It is also well documented from large randomised trials in cervical and anal cancer that the pelvic nodes can be treated "en bloc" with acceptable toxicity, a major problem with large-scale surgical dissection.

Metastatic disease

Treatment results in patients with distant metastatic disease are currently disappointing. Chemotherapy is the mainstay, often in combination with other modalities, but effective agents are lacking. Overall prognosis is poor and response to therapy is affected by age and performance status. Most of the limited data available come from small non-randomised series

Chapter 3

which differ widely in their patient selection, treatment doses and schedules. In the absence of randomised clinical trials, there is no consensus on the optimal chemotherapy regimen. In a recent survey of type of chemotherapy used in advanced penile cancer by urologists and oncologists in the UK, seven different single and multi-agent chemotherapy regimens were identified. Combination chemotherapy appears to be superior to single agent treatment but results in increased toxicity [28]. The agents with the best response include 5-fluorouracil, bleomycin, methotrexate and cisplatin. In the largest multi-institutional prospective clinical trial to be carried out in penile cancer, the SWOG group reported a 32.5% overall response rate to cisplatin in combination with methotrexate and bleomycin in 40 patients with locally advanced or metastatic penile cancer. However, a cautionary finding was five treatment-related deaths and a life-threatening toxic episode in six other patients [29] **(IIb/B)**. An alternative promising combination is vincristine, bleomycin and methotrexate for which a response rate of 54% has been reported with apparently less toxicity than the cisplatin-based regimen [30]. The EAU recommends this adjuvant treatment as a 12-week course, given once a week in the outpatient setting [5]. Docetaxel is another newer agent currently being investigated by the SWOG group.

For now, the precise role of chemotherapy either alone or as part of integrated therapy for advanced penile cancer remains unclear and more effective agents with minimal toxicity need to be developed.

Conclusions

Several questions in the management of lymph nodes in patients with penile cancer need to be answered. Research evidence in the form of large, well designed, multi-centre randomised controlled trials is urgently needed so that these currently controversial issues can be addressed and patients can be offered effective evidence-based treatments for this rare and still relatively poorly understood disease.

Recommendations	Evidence level

What is the importance of lymph node status?

- Inguinal lymph node status is the most important prognostic factor for long-term survival in penile cancer. — III/B
- Multiple (greater than two) or bilateral node involvement and extracapsular tumour are adverse prognostic features. — III/B

What is the management of patients with palpable lymph nodes?

- Approximately 50% have palpable nodes at presentation of which half are due to tumour involvement. — III/B
- Routine early inguinal lymphadenectomy is beneficial in this group with average five-year survival rates of 60%. — III/B

Lymphadenectomy or surveillance in patients with impalpable lymph nodes?

- Only 20% have histologically positive nodes. — III/B
- Routine prophylactic inguinal lymphadenectomy potentially over treats 80% of cases.
- Overall evidence suggests an improvement in survival in patients offered early versus late lymphadenectomy. — III/B
- Stratification of patients into risk groups based on histological features of the primary tumour has enabled management strategies to be developed. — IV/C

Which is the best surveillance modality for the inguinal regions?

- Physical examination alone may be inaccurate, with a sensitivity of 82% and a specificity of 79%. — III/B
- USS +/- FNA is the recommended investigation in patients who are clinically node-negative but at high risk of occult metastases. — III/B
- Dynamic sentinel lymph node biopsy is a promising and reliable technique for the detection of early lymph node metastases (reported sensitivity 80%). — III/B

What are the complications of inguinal lymphadenectomy?

- Classical "radical" inguinal lymphadenectomy is associated with a complication rate of nearly 85%. — III/B
- A "modified" block dissection technique has been shown to minimise morbidity without compromising tumour clearance. — III/B

Chapter 3

Recommendations *continued:*	Evidence level

What is the role of radiotherapy?

- Five-year survival rates in patients with inguinal metastases treated with surgery are superior to those treated with radiotherapy. — IIb/B
- Palliative radiotherapy can be offered to patients with bulky or fixed inoperable nodes.
- Adjuvant radiotherapy is recommended in patients with three or more positive nodes or extracapsular involvement. — III/B

How should the iliac nodes be managed?

- Patients with two or more positive inguinal nodes or extracapsular invasion have a 20%-30% risk of pelvic nodal involvement. — IIa-III/B
- Five-year survival for patients with positive pelvic nodes is around 10%. — III/B
- In selected patients, pelvic lymphadenectomy can improve loco-regional control.

What is the role of chemotherapy in metastatic disease?

- Treatment results in patients with distant metastatic disease are currently disappointing.
- In the absence of randomised clinical trials, there is no consensus on the optimal chemotherapy regimen. — III/B
- Combination chemotherapy appears to be superior to single agent treatment.

References

1. Office for National Statistics. Cancer Trends in England and Wales, 1950-1999.
2. Horenblas S, van Tinteren H. Squamous cell carcinoma of the penis. IV. Prognostic factors of survival: analysis of tumor, nodes and metastasis classification system. *J Urol* 1994; 151(5): 1239-1243.
3. Lopes A, Hidalgo GS, Kowalski LP, Torloni H, Rossi BM, Fonseca FP. Prognostic factors in carcinoma of the penis: multivariate analysis of 145 patients treated with amputation and lymphadenectomy. *J Urol* 1996; 156(5): 1637-1642.
4. Srinivas V, Morse MJ, Herr HW, Sogani PC, Whitmore WF, Jr. Penile cancer: relation of extent of nodal metastasis to survival. *J Urol* 1987; 137(5): 880-882.
5. Algaba F, Horenblas S, Pizzocaro-Luigi PG, Solsona E, Windahl T. EAU guidelines on penile cancer. *Eur Urol* 2002; 42(3): 199-203.
6. Ekstrom T, Edsmyr F. Cancer of the penis; a clinical study of 229 cases. *Acta Chir Scand* 1958; 115(1-2): 25-45.
7. Ravi R. Prophylactic lymphadenectomy vs observation vs inguinal biopsy in node-negative patients with invasive carcinoma of the penis. *Jpn J Clin Oncol* 1993; 23(1): 53-58.
8. Ornellas AA, Seixas AL, Marota A, Wisnescky A, Campos F, de Moraes JR. Surgical treatment of invasive squamous cell carcinoma of the penis: retrospective analysis of 350 cases. *J Urol* 1994; 151(5): 1244-1249.
9. Fraley EE, Zhang G, Manivel C, Niehans GA. The role of ilioinguinal lymphadenectomy and significance of histological differentiation in treatment of carcinoma of the penis. *J Urol* 1989; 142(6): 1478-1482.
10. Johnson DE, Lo RK. Complications of groin dissection in penile cancer. Experience with 101 lymphadenectomies. *Urology* 1984; 24(4): 312-314.
11. McDougal WS, Kirchner FK, Jr., Edwards RH, Killion LT. Treatment of carcinoma of the penis: the case for primary lymphadenectomy. *J Urol* 1986; 136(1): 38-41.

12. Horenblas S, van Tinteren H, Delemarre JF, Moonen LM, Lustig V, Kroger R. Squamous cell carcinoma of the penis: accuracy of tumor, nodes and metastasis classification system, and role of lymphangiography, computerized tomography scan and fine needle aspiration cytology. *J Urol* 1991; 146(5): 1279-1283.

13. Horenblas S, van Tinteren H, Delemarre JF, Moonen LM, Lustig V, van Waardenburg EW. Squamous cell carcinoma of the penis. III. Treatment of regional lymph nodes. *J Urol* 1993; 149(3): 492-497.

14. Horenblas S. Lymphadenectomy for squamous cell carcinoma of the penis. Part 1: diagnosis of lymph node metastasis. *BJU Int* 2001; 88(5): 467-472.

15. Cabanas RM. An approach for the treatment of penile carcinoma. *Cancer* 1977; 39(2): 456-466.

16. Tanis PJ, Lont AP, Meinhardt W, Olmos RA, Nieweg OE, Horenblas S. Dynamic sentinel node biopsy for penile cancer: reliability of a staging technique. *J Urol* 2002; 168(1): 76-80.

17. Akduman B, Fleshner NE, Ehrlich L, Klotz L. Early experience in intermediate-risk penile cancer with sentinel node identification using the gamma probe. *Urology* 2001; 58(1): 65-68.

18. Lont AP, Horenblas S, Tanis PJ, Gallee MP, van Tinteren H, Nieweg OE. Management of clinically node negative penile carcinoma: improved survival after the introduction of dynamic sentinel node biopsy. *J Urol* 2003; 170(3): 783-786.

19. Bevan-Thomas R, Slaton JW, Pettaway CA. Contemporary morbidity from lymphadenectomy for penile squamous cell carcinoma: the MD Anderson Cancer Center Experience. *J Urol* 2002; 167(4): 1638-1642.

20. Catalona WJ. Modified inguinal lymphadenectomy for carcinoma of the penis with preservation of saphenous veins: technique and preliminary results. *J Urol* 1988; 140(2): 306-310.

21. Jacobellis U. Modified radical inguinal lymphadenectomy for carcinoma of the penis: technique and results. *J Urol* 2003; 169(4): 1349-1352.

22. Staubitz WJ, Lent MH, Oberkircher OJ. Carcinoma of the penis. *Cancer* 1955; 8(2): 371-378.

23. Murrell DS, Williams JL. Radiotherapy in the treatment of carcinoma of the penis. *Br J Urol* 1965; 37: 211-222.

24. Pow-Sang JE, Benavente V, Pow-Sang JM, Pow-Sang M. Bilateral ilioinguinal lymph node dissection in the management of cancer of the penis. *Semin Surg Oncol* 1990; 6(4): 241-242.

25. de Kernion JB, Tynberg P, Persky L, Fegen JP. Proceedings: carcinoma of the penis. *Cancer* 1973; 32(5): 1256-1262.

26. Rose PG, Bundy BN, Watkins EB, Thigpen JT, Deppe G, Maiman MA, *et al.* Concurrent cisplatin-based radiotherapy and chemotherapy for locally advanced cervical cancer. *N Engl J Med* 1999; 340(15): 1144-1153.

27. Epidermoid anal cancer: results from the UKCCCR randomised trial of radiotherapy alone versus radiotherapy, 5-fluorouracil, and mitomycin. UKCCCR Anal Cancer Trial Working Party. UK Co-ordinating Committee on Cancer Research. *Lancet* 1996; 348(9034): 1049-1054.

28. Culkin DJ, Beer TM. Advanced penile carcinoma. *J Urol* 2003; 170(2 Pt 1): 359-365.

29. Haas GP, Blumenstein BA, Gagliano RG, Russell CA, Rivkin SE, Culkin DJ, *et al.* Cisplatin, methotrexate and bleomycin for the treatment of carcinoma of the penis: a Southwest Oncology Group study. *J Urol* 1999; 161(6): 1823-1825.

30. Pizzocaro G, Piva L. Adjuvant and neoadjuvant vincristine, bleomycin, and methotrexate for inguinal metastases from squamous cell carcinoma of the penis. *Acta Oncol* 1988; 27(6b): 823-824.

Chapter 3

Chapter 3

Chapter 4

Testicular microlithiasis: a sinister condition?

Johan Poulsen MD FEBU, Consultant Urologist [1,2]
Paul S Sidhu MRCP FRCR, Consultant Radiologist [2]
Mette Holm MD, Specialist Registrar, Urology [3]

1 AALBORG UNIVERSITY HOSPITAL, DENMARK
2 KING'S COLLEGE HOSPITAL, LONDON, UK
3 DEPARTMENT OF GROWTH AND REPRODUCTION,
RIGSHOSPITALET, COPENHAGEN, DENMARK

Introduction

In tissues such as thyroid and mammary glands, microcalcifications detected on radiological examinations are known to be associated with an increased risk for cancer. Earlier studies have also demonstrated this connection in testicular cancer [1] (III/B). Due to the radiation side effects, testicular x-rays have been kept to a minimum. Ultrasound examination, on the contrary, is often used and "new" findings of testicular microcalcifications or microlithiasis have been noticed as well as a possible connection to germ cell cancer. In this chapter we will focus on data related to this possible association.

Testicular cancer and CIS

Testicular cancer mainly affects younger men. The incidence varies from country to country and has been steadily increasing over the past few decades. In the decade between 1940 and 1950, the incidence among American men was estimated at 2.88 per 100,000 [2], increasing to 4.5 per 100,000 in 1990 [3]. Denmark has one of the world's highest incidences of testicular cancers, estimated at about six cases per 100,000 men [4]. The risk of testicular cancer is increased in patients with undescended testes (2%-4%), contralateral cancer (5%), extra gonadal germ cell cancer (up to 40%) and in cases of intersex [5] (IIb/B).

Testicular cancer arises from carcinoma *in situ* (CIS) cells on the basal membrane of the seminiferous tubules. CIS is thought to develop in foetal life gaining its invasive potential only after puberty. In men diagnosed with CIS, the risk of developing invasive carcinoma within five years is 50% [6], while the remainder probably will all develop a tumour after a longer period. With the documented progression of CIS into invasive tumour, its prevalence declines with age, becoming minimal after 50 years [6] (IIb/B).

Although the "cure rate" for testicular cancer approaches 90%-95%, the morbidity associated with the radiotherapy and chemotherapy regimens remains.

If detected, the pre-cancerous CIS lesion can be treated by testicular irradiation (in bilateral cases or in a solitary testicle) or by orchidectomy [7] (III/B). The ideal situation thus would be to diagnose and treat CIS. This is a rare event as CIS is asymptomatic.

Chapter 4

Testicular microlithiasis

Testicular microlithiasis (TM) (Figure 1) has recently been found to be associated with germ cell tumours and CIS [8,9]. On high-resolution ultrasound TM is seen as multiple small echogenic foci within the testicular parenchyma without associated acoustic shadowing. One definition for TM suggests that at least five, 1-3mm foci should be seen on one testicular image using a high resolution 7-10 MHz linear array transducer [10,11]. TM can be seen in prepubertal boys and in adults as a localised lesion in one testicle or dispersed in one or both testicles. CIS lesions however, are almost never diagnosed in prepubertal boys. We will therefore focus on TM in adults only.

Among 198 healthy volunteers TM was found in 1.5% [12], while the prevalence of TM in the largest series of 1504 healthy young men was 5.6%. None of these 84 men had a testicular tumour and markers were normal in all [13]. The authors' comparison of cancer incidence with the prevalence of TM is mistaken. The comparison should be between lifetime risk for testicular cancer and prevalence of TM (supposed to be a risk factor for CIS) [14] **(IV/C)**. However, testicular biopsies were not obtained and long-term follow-up of the TM-affected testicles has not as yet been published in these series.

In several papers, where a testicular ultrasound examination was performed for clinical reasons, a testicular tumour has been reported in 23%-73% of men with microlithiasis [8,9,15-18]. Among patients without microlithiasis, the frequency of a testicular tumour was 2.1%-6% only [9,17]. The prevalence of microlithiasis in testicles contralateral to cancer is also found to be markedly higher than in normal men (14%-16.9%), and these testicles are known to be at an increased risk for CIS [12,19,20] **(IIb/B)**.

The odds ratio for CIS in a patient with contralateral TM is 28.6 and the frequency of microlithiasis significantly higher in testicles with contralateral CIS compared to those with a normal echo pattern. To date, a total number of 12 patients with TM have been reported to develop testicular cancer over an observational period of six months to eleven years (Table 1) [9,15,17,18,26].

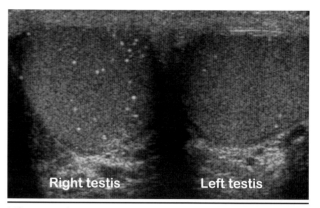

Figure 1. Transverse ultrasound image of the testicles using a 10MHz linear array transducer. The right testis demonstrates multiple foci of high echogenicity in keeping with microlithiasis, whereas on the left there are fewer areas of microlithiasis demonstrated.

The presumption is that all these patients had CIS before the development of tumour; in other words at the time they were diagnosed with TM. This association of TM with the pre-invasive precursor of testicular germ cell neoplasia, carcinoma *in situ*, was initially reported by Kragel *et al* [21] and several years later by Lenz *et al* [22]. However, the prevalence of CIS in patients with TM has only been investigated to a limited extent. In a series of 11 infertile patients with TM, biopsy revealed CIS in two cases (18%)[12]. Among 64 testicles contralateral to cancer, nine had TM, and seven of these were diagnosed with CIS in that testicle (78%). Conversely, in a series of 12 asymptomatic patients with TM, eight underwent a testicular biopsy of which all showed a normal histological pattern without any neoplasia or CIS [23]. In the original study first describing TM, biopsy showed sertoli cell only (SCO) and no signs of CIS or cancer [24].

When evaluating these data however, it is necessary to realise that the diagnosis of testicular CIS depends on good quality histological samples. The biopsies have to contain at least 30 seminiferous tubules and be handled very gently. The fixative used should be Stieve's or Bouin's solution, and never formalin (which destroys the testicular parenchyma). Furthermore, the diagnostic security can be increased by immunostaining with Placenta like Alkaline Phosphatase (PLAP).

Table 1. Summary of 12 cases undergoing an ultrasound examination, with multiple echogenic areas demonstrated in the testis (considered to be testicular microlithiasis). These cases reported in the literature have, after an observational period, progressed to a testicular tumour.

Age (years) at first US	Reasons for investigation	Testis affected with TM	Testicular volume	Interval to tumour detection	Histology	Reference
32	Infertility and left side cryptorchism repaired age 11 years	Right	Atrophic	10 months	Embryonal carcinoma	Salisz et al 1990 [38]
17	Discrepancy in testicular volume	Bilateral	Normal	4 years	Yolk sac tumour	McEniff et al 1996 [39]
21	Testicular pain and haematospermia	Left	Not reported	3 years	Mixed germ cell	Winter et al 1996 [9]
25	Testicular enlargement	Bilateral	Not reported	16 months	Mixed germ cell	Frush et al 1996 [40]
29	Seminoma right testis	Left	Atrophic	11 years	Seminoma	Gooding 1997 [41]
47	Testicular pain	Bilateral	Right atrophic, left normal	6 months	Seminoma right/CIS left	Golash et al 2001 [42]
Not reported	Follow-up. Left orchidectomy for embryonal tumour 10 years earlier Bilateral childhood cryptorchism	Bilateral	Atrophic	35 months	Teratoma and seminoma	Derogee et al 2001 [17]
29	Bilateral atrophic testis	Bilateral	Atrophic	2 years	Seminoma	Otite et al 2001 [15]
34	Follow-up after extra gonadal germ cell tumour	Right	Atrophic	4 years	Seminoma	Otite et al 2001 [15]
31	Follow-up after left seminoma	Right	Atrophic	3 years	Seminoma	Kaveggia et al 1996 [26]
Not reported	Follow-up for bilateral TM Previous cryptorchism	Unknown	Atrophic	4 years	Seminoma	Sibert et al 2002 [43]
25	Hydrocele	Bilateral	Normal	1 year	Seminoma	de Ryke et al 2003 [44]

US=ultrasound; TM=testicular microlithiasis; CIS=carcinoma in situ

Chapter 4

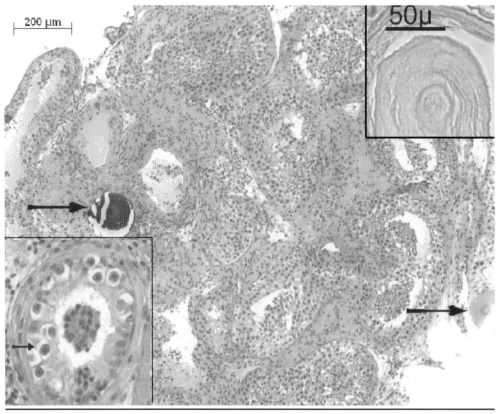

Figure 2. Haematoxylin and eosin-stained testicular biopsy showing impaired spermato-genesis and microliths (large arrows).
Inserts: upper right=higher magnification of microliths; lower left=tubule with CIS cells.

When these criteria are fulfilled, the number of false negative biopsies is judged to be 0.3%-0.5% [25]. Diagnoses of CIS by means of semen samples are so far disappointing. It would seem that the key to understanding the significance of TM is dependent on future larger series investigating the relationship between ultrasound and histology. In general, testicles reported with TM and associated CIS are small [12,15,26,27] **(IIb/B and III/B)**.

Microliths

Microliths can be seen on histological examination of testicular parenchyma [14] as spherical bodies with a central calcified core surrounded by concentric layers of more or less calcified hyaline substance. The size of microliths varies from very small and easily missed to large bodies filling the entire lumen of a seminiferous tubule. On HE staining they can be basophilic or eosinophilic.

Among 218 testicles contralateral to cancer, carcinoma *in situ* was seen in 8.7% of biopsies and 6% had microliths (Figure 2). In another histological series, microliths were diagnosed in 38% of biopsies with CIS, but only in 2.1% of testicular biopsies without CIS [28]. It is presumed that microliths on histology shows as TM on ultrasound if the size and numbers are large enough to be detected by a high frequency ultrasound transducer. However, other phenomena in the tissue might be reflected as TM. For instance, an inexperienced examiner may in certain projections mistake the rete testis for TM.

Variations of ultrasonographical TM

The currently accepted definition of TM is the presence of at least five non-enhancing echogenic foci, 1-3mm in diameter, seen simultaneously on one image of the testicular parenchyma.

The main difference between histological microlithiasis and TM seems to be a ten-fold difference in size [29] **(III/B)** (Figure 3), but whether the histologically proven microliths are identical to those 1-3mm echogenic points on the ultrasound scan remains to be investigated.

Some authors describe different types of echogenic areas on a background of differing tissue patterns on the ultrasound image, where the texture pattern is suggestive of the presence of CIS [22,30] **(IIb/B)**.

In some series, TM is considered present with as few as three [17], five [10,11,13], or as many as ten foci on the same cross-sectional image of the testicular parenchyma [12].

Other echogenic foci

Obviously some intra-testicular calcifications occurring in association with germ cell tumours do have another pathogenesis. They may be caused by focal necrosis, trauma or calcific foci in mixed germ cell tumours, especially teratomas [31,32]. Also, various benign conditions have been associated with testicular calcifications (epidermoid cysts, benign cystic teratomas, testicular multicystic dysplasia, ectopic adrenal nests, testicular sarcoidosis, tuberculosis, haematomas and infarction) [33].

The significance of TM remains unclear. Comparing figures of retrospective to prospective studies is probably not very informative. Retrospective review of ultrasound images leads to interpretational difficulties

Chapter 4

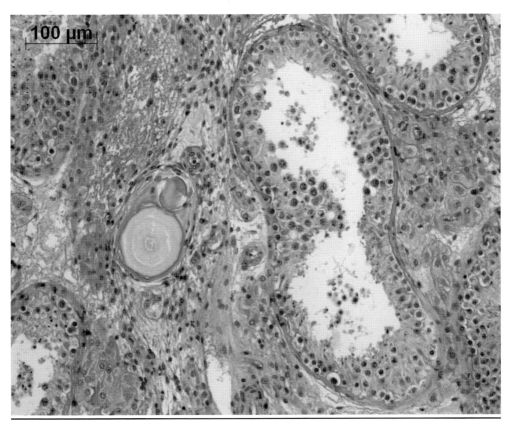

Figure 3. Testicular microlith filling the lumen of a completely atrophic seminiferous tubule.

and valuable information may not have been recorded. Whether the current definition of TM is the correct one, or irregular texture pattern without calcification also ought to be included, remains a question.

The only way to clarify whether TM represents a herald of CIS is to either perform regular follow-up of patients with TM or to obtain biopsies in all patients with TM which over a long period would establish the exact numerical risk of harbouring CIS in patients with TM.

Currently, the management of the patient with TM is confused. Some authors recommend that in patients with TM, routine biopsy should be performed [12,34] **(IIb/B and III/B)**, and ultrasound examinations at 6-12 monthly intervals should be offered [12,35] **(IIb/B and III/B)**; others suggest some clinical surveillance [36] **(III/B)**, and no follow-up needed at all also has been proposed[13] **(IIb/B)**.

At King's College Hospital, London, patients with TM have been offered an ultrasound scan on a yearly basis [37].

Conclusions

There seems to be no doubt that TM is related to testicular tumour and CIS. The question is to what extent the risk for CIS/cancer is increased among men with TM. Prevalence studies document the existence of TM or irregular texture pattern in 1.5%-8.1% of healthy young men, in whom the lifetime risk for testicular cancer, i.e. prevalence of CIS in high risk areas as Denmark, is a little less than 1%. Roughly half of the men with testicular cancer demonstrate TM in that testicle at the time of diagnosis.

For the time being, while the results of ongoing studies are awaited, it may be recommended to include any possible patients in these studies. If this is not possible the patient should be informed that at present there seems to be a somewhat increased risk for carcinoma *in situ* and later, testicular cancer. Bilateral testicular biopsies should be considered, especially if other risk factors (as mentioned) are present in a man belonging to the relevant age group for CIS (18-55 years of age).

Recommendations	Evidence level
◆ Testicular carcinoma *in situ* is related to subsequent carcinoma formation.	IIa/B
◆ TM is related to CIS in patients with testicular symptoms or complaints.	III/B
◆ TM is related to CIS in patients with a history of testicular non descent.	III/B
◆ TM is related to CIS in patients with testicular atrophy.	III/B
◆ TM is related to CIS in patients, who have had contralateral testicular cancer.	IIb/B
◆ TM has no relation to testicular CIS in asymptomatic young men.	IV/C

Chapter 4

References

1. Würster and Menges. Virchows Arch. *A Path Anat and Histol* 1977; 374: 45-62.

2. Dixon FJ, Moore RA. Tumors of the male sex organs. In: *Atlas of Tumor Pathology*. Section VIII, Fasciles 31b and 32. Armed forces Institute of Pathology, Washington DC, 1952: 127.

3. Feuer EJ, Brown LM, Kaplan RS. Testis. In: *SEER Cancer Statistics Review 1973-1990*. Miller BA, Gloeckler LA, Hankey BF, *et al*, Eds. National Institutes of Health, Bethesda, MD.

4. Osterlind A. Diverging trends in incidence and mortality of testicular cancer in Denmark 1943-1982. *Br J Cancer* 1986; 53: 501-506.

5. Müller J, Skakkebæk NE, Ritzen EM, Plöen L, Petersen KE. Carcinoma *in situ* of the testis in children with 45, X/46, XY gonadal dysgenesis. *J Pediatr* 1985; 106: 431-436.

6. Skakkebæk NE, Berthelsen JG, Givercman A, Müller J. Carcinoma *in situ* of the testis: a review. In: *Morphological basis of human reproductive function*. Spera G. Kretser DM, Eds. Plenum Press, New York and London, 1987: 25-34.

7. Steele RJ. Neoplasma of the testis. In: *Campbell's Urology*, 8th Edition. Walsh, Retik, Vaughan Wein, Eds. Elsevier Science, London, New York, 2002: 2879-2880.

8. Ganem JP, Workman KR, Shaban SF. Testicular microlithiasis is associated with testicular pathology. *Urology* 1999; 53: 209-213.

9. Winter TC III, Zunkel DE, Mack LA. Testicular carcinoma in a patient with previously demonstrated microlithiasis. *J Urol* 1996; 155: 648.

10. Janzen D, Mathieson J, Marsh J, *et al*. Testicular microlithiasis: sonography and clinical features. *Am J Roentgenol* 1992; 158: 1057-1062.

11. Hobarth K, Susani M, Szabo N. Incidence of testicular microlithiasis. *Urology* 1992; 40: 464-466.

12. Von Ekardstein S, Tsakmakidis G, Kamischke A, Rolf C, Nieschlag E. Sonographic testicular microlithiasis as an indicator of premalignant conditions in normal and infertile men. *Journal of Andrology* 2001; 22: 818-824.

13. Peterson AC, Bauman JM, Light DE, McMann LP, Costabile RA. The prevalence of testicular microlithiasis in an asymptomatic population of men 18 to 35 years old. *J Urol* 2001; 166: 2061-2064.

14. Holm M, Rajpert-De Meyts E, Daugaard C, Skakkebæk NE. The prevalence of testicular microlithiasis in an asymptomatic population of men 18-35 years old. *J Urol* 2002; 168: 1108.

15. Otite U, Webb JAW, Oliver RTD, Badenoch DF, Narguud VH. Testicular microlithiasis: is it a benign condition with malignant potential. *Eur Urol* 2001; 40: 538-542.

16. Hobarth K, Szabo N, Klinger HC, *et al*. Sonographic appearances of testicular microlithiasis. *Eur Urol* 1993; 24: 251-255.

17. Derogee M, Bevers RFM, Prins HJ, Jones TGN, Elbers FH, Boon TA. Testicular microlithiasis, a premalignant condition: prevalence, histopathologic findings and relation to testicular tumor. *Urology* 2001; 57: 1133-1137.

18. Ikinger U, Wurster K, Terwey B. Microcalcifications in testicular malignancy. *Urology* 1982; 19: 525-529.

19. Bach AM, Hann LE, Shi W, Giess CS, Yoo HH, Sheinfeld J, Thaler P. Is there an increased incidence of contralateral testicular cancer in patients with intratesticular microlithiasis? *Am J Roentgenol* 2003; 180: 497-500.

20. Holm M, Hoei-Hansen CE, Rajpert- De Meyts E, Skakkebæk NE. Increased risk of carcinoma *in situ* in patients with testicular germ cell cancer with ultrasonic microlithiasis in the contralateral testicle. *J Urol* 2003; 170: 1163-1167.

21. Kragel, PJ Delveccio, D. Orlando R, *et al*. Ultrasonographic findings of testicular findings of testicular microlithiasis associated with intratubular germ cell neoplasia. *Urology* 1991; 37: 66-68.

22. Lenz S, Giwercman A, Skakkebæk NE, Bruun E, Frimodt-Møller C. Ultrasound in detection of early neoplasia of the testis. *Int J Androl* 1987; 10: 187-190.

23. Schering L, Kvist E, Rasmussen SG, Wahlin AB. Testicular microlithiasis - are biopsy and follow-up necessary? *Ugeskrift for laeger* 2002; 164: 2041-2045.

24. Doherty FJ, Mulling TL, Sant GR, Drinkwater MA, Ucci AAJ. Testicular microlithiasis. a unique sonographic appearance. *J Ultrasound Med* 1987; 6: 389-392.

25. Dieckmann KP, Loy V. False negative biopsies for the diagnosis of testicular intraepithelial neoplasia (TIN) - an update. *Eur Urol* 2003; 43: 516-521.

26. Kaveggia FF, Stassman MJ, Apfelbach GL, Hatch JL, Wirlanen GW. Diffuse testicular microlithiasis associated with intra tubular germ cell, neoplasia and seminoma. *Urology* 1996; 48: 794-796.

27. Giwercman A, von der Maase H, Rorth M, Skakkebæk NE. Semen quality in testicular tumour and CIS in the contralateral testis. *Lancet* 1993; 341: 384-385.

28. Kang J-L, Raj pert-De Meyts E, Giwercman A, Skakkebæk NE. The association of testicular carcinoma *in situ* with intra tubular micro calcifications. *J Urol Pathol* 1994; 2: 235-242.

29. Freeman A, Rowbotham C, Parkinson MC. Letter to the editor. *J Urol* 2003; 169: 1474.

30. Lenz S, Giwercman A, Elsborg A, Cohr K-H, Jelnes JE, Carlsen E, Skakkebæk NE. Ultrasonic texture and size in 444 men from the general population. Correction to semen quality. *Eur Urol* 1993; 24: 231-238.

31. Grantham G, Charboneau JW, James EM, Kirschling RJ, Kvols CK, Segura JW, *et al*. Testicular neoplasma: 29 tumours studied by high resolution ultrasound. *Radiology* 1985; 157: 775-780.

32. Krone MD, Carrol MD. Scrotal ultrasound. *Radiol Clin North Am* 1985; 23: 121-139.

33. Bushby LH, Miller FNAC, Rosario S, Clarke JL, Sidhu PS. Pictorial review, scrotal calcifications: ultrasound appearances, distributions and aetiology. *Br J Radiol* 2002; 75: 283-288.

34. Wegner H.E, Hubotter A, Andresen R, Miller K. Testicular microlithiasis and concomitant testicular intra epithelial neoplasia. *Int Urol Nephrol* 1998; 30: 313-315.

Chapter 4

35. Cast JE, Nelson WN, Early AS, Bryani S, Cooksey G, Warnock NG, Breen DJ. Testicular microlithiasis: prevalence and tumour risk in a population referred for scrotal sonography. *Am J Roentgenol* 2000; 175: 1703-1706.

36. Bach AM, Hanu LE, Hadar O, Shi W, Yoo HH, Giess CS, Scheinfeld J, Thaler H. Testicular microlithiasis: what is its association with testicular cancer? *Radiology* 2001; 220: 70-75.

37. Miller FNAC, Sidhu PS. Does testicular microlithiasis matter? A review. *Clin Radiol* 2002, 57: 883-890.

38. Salisz JA, Goldman KA. Testicular calcifications and neoplasia in a patient treated for sub fertility. *Urology* 1990; 36; 557-560.

39. McEniff N, Doherty F, Katz J, Schrager CS, Klauber G. Yolk sac tumour of the testis discovered on a routine annual sonogram on a boy with testicular microlithiasis. *Am J Roentgenol* 1995; 164; 971-972.

40. Frush DP, Kliewer MA, Madden JF. Testicular microlithiasis and subsequent development of metastatic germ cell. *Am J Roentgenol* 1996; 167; 889-890.

41. Gooding GA, Detection of testicular microlithiasis by sonography. *Am J Roentgenol* 1997; 168; 281-282.

42. Golash A, Parker J, Ennis O, Jenkins BJ. The interval of development of testicular carcinoma in a patient with previously demonstrated testicular microlithiasis. *J Urol* 2000; 163; 239.

43. Siebert R.D, Roset F, Dunet F, Staerman F, Grise P. Testicular microlithiasis and cancer of the testis. *Progres en urologie* 2002; 12; 500-503.

44. Lawrentschuk N, Stephen J, Brough S, de Ryke J. Testicular mircolithiasis: a case report and review of the literature. *ANZ Journal of Surgery* 2003; 73; 364-366.

Chapter 5

Surgery versus chemotherapy for high risk NSGCT: why surgery?

Richard S Foster MD

Professor of Urology

INDIANA UNIVERSITY MEDICAL CENTER, INDIANAPOLIS, USA

High risk clinical stage I nonseminoma

After radical orchidectomy for non-seminomatous testis cancer, patients undergo clinical staging. Clinical staging studies include CT scans of the abdomen and chest and determination of serum alpha fetoprotein and beta HCG. If the CT scans show no evidence of metastatic disease, and if tumour markers have normalised or are falling according to half lives of 1½ days for beta HCG and five days for alpha fetoprotein, the patient is termed clinical stage I. It is well recognised that approximately 30% of clinical stage I patients in fact have occult metastatic disease, usually, but not always, to the retroperitoneal lymph nodes.

A prospective study of clinical stage I non-seminoma patients using surveillance identified risk factors in the orchidectomy specimen predictive of occult metastatic disease [1]. These factors included vascular invasion, lymphatic invasion, presence of embryonal carcinoma, and absence of yolk sac elements. Patients with all of these elements had a risk of occult metastatic disease of around 50% as opposed to the 30% level in all patients with non-seminoma.

Many confirmatory studies from around the world have verified that these factors are indeed important [2,3]. Currently, most clinicians treating these patients use vascular and lymphatic invasion as the primary indicator of high risk disease. It is fair to state that if patients have a high amount of embryonal carcinoma and vascular/lymphatic invasion, the risk of relapse on a surveillance protocol is around 40%-50%, and therefore, these factors are accepted as indicative of high risk disease **(II/B)**.

Chance for cure

Though prospective randomised studies have not been conducted comparing the primary methods of management of patients with clinical stage I non-seminoma, it appears that the chance for cure is around 99% regardless of the method of management chosen **(III/B)**. Currently, the methods used to manage these patients include surveillance with standard dose chemotherapy at relapse, nerve-sparing retroperitoneal lymph node dissection (RPLND), and primary chemotherapy which usually consists of two courses of bleomycin, etoposide, and cisplatin (BEP). Individual series of patients managed with each of these methods of management has shown that in the short-term the chance for cure is around 99%[1,3,4]. Whether or not there are differences in late relapse between initial surgical treatment of metastasis (nerve-sparing RPLND) and medical methods of management (surveillance, primary chemotherapy) is unclear. There is at least a theoretical foundation to suspect that initial surgical treatment would yield a lower probability of late relapse but there is no hard data to confirm this supposition.

Hence, in clinical stage I disease, patients can be assured that the chance for cure is very high regardless of the method of management. Since chance for cure is equal, choosing between methods of management is contingent upon individual patient desires and potential side effects of therapy.

Why nerve-sparing RPLND?

The rationale behind proceeding with nerve-sparing RPLND is predicated upon a unique aspect of testis cancer biology. Testis cancer is not only very chemosensitive it is also "surgical sensitive". Fully 50%-75% of patients with metastatic testis cancer to retroperitoneal lymph nodes can be cured merely by the surgical removal of these lymph nodes [3] **(III/B)**. This is certainly rare in the general population of all cancer patients with metastasis as most patients with lymphatic metastasis have coexistent occult systemic metastasis. Therefore, the surgical removal of lymph nodes in the general population of all cancer patients is not usually curative. This singular fact makes testis cancer unique.

Therefore, nerve-sparing RPLND is a very effective "single agent". A new chemotherapeutic agent with the capability of curing 50%-75% of patients would indeed be a major advance in medical therapy of cancer. However, nerve-sparing RPLND must stand another test; it must have a low enough morbidity to justify its use.

In experienced hands, nerve-sparing RPLND is a procedure of about two hours in length. Transfusion is not required and, with prospective nerve-sparing, emission and ejaculation are preserved in greater than

99% of patients. At Indiana University, the average hospitalisation is three days and return to full physical activity occurs in four to six weeks. Because testis cancer is a disease of young men, recovery is generally rapid and return to full physical activity usually occurs prior to four to six weeks.

The acute surgical morbidity from the procedure consists of an approximate 1% chance of developing a small bowel obstruction due to adhesions and a 3% -5% chance of developing an incisional hernia [5]. Because this is a relatively short procedure performed in healthy patients, wound infections are uncommon and essentially, the morbidity of the procedure is that of a laparotomy.

Therefore, nerve-sparing RPLND is an effective single agent curing approximately 50%-75% of those with lymphatic metastasis and is associated with low morbidity. Additionally, the follow-up after nerve-sparing RPLND is easy and straightforward consisting of periodic chest x-rays and marker determinations for a period of two years. Recurrence of disease beyond two years from the date of initial surgery is extremely rare.

Arguments against chemotherapy

As noted above, if patients with so-called high risk disease are treated with two courses of bleomycin, etoposide, and cisplatin, 99% are cured in the short-term. Because around 50% of patients who have high risk disease in fact were cured with orchidectomy alone and have no distant metastatic disease, 50% of patients treated with primary chemotherapy receive therapy from which they derive no benefit. If the morbidity of administration of two courses of BEP were negligible, this exposure of 50% of patients with no metastatic disease to chemotherapy would not be problematic. Hence, the short- and long-term morbidity of chemotherapy becomes a very pertinent issue.

The short-term morbidity of testis cancer chemotherapy has certainly decreased from the mid 1970s to the current time. Effective anti-emetics and growth factors have decreased the short-term morbidity to the point that standard BEP chemotherapy is now administered as an outpatient.

However, there have been many recent studies investigating the long-term morbidity of testis cancer chemotherapy. It is recognised that BEP chemotherapy has an effect on spermatogenesis in the contralateral testis. Studies performed on patients who received three or four courses of chemotherapy have shown that although some patients regain complete spermatogenesis, some are rendered azoospermic and some have decreased sperm quality when semen analyses are done one or two years after chemotherapy [6]. Though claims have been made that two courses of BEP have no effect on spermatogenesis, adequate numbers of patients have not been studied pre- and post-chemotherapy in order to prove no difference [7]. Though there is evidence that many of the side effects of testis cancer chemotherapy are dose-related, some do not appear to be dose-related [8,9]. Regarding spermatogenesis, it is likely that a greater difference exists between no courses of chemotherapy and two courses of chemotherapy compared to two courses of chemotherapy versus three courses of chemotherapy. Since many patients with testis cancer have impaired spermatogenesis at presentation, it is highly likely that spermatogenesis is affected in some patients who receive only two courses of chemotherapy.

Other recent studies have examined long-term effects of testis cancer chemotherapy on cardiovascular disease. Studies from The Netherlands have identified abnormal blood lipids and a higher probability of a cardiovascular event in patients treated with testis cancer chemotherapy [10]. More recently, a study from the UK confirmed this cardiovascular effect and indicated that some of the side effects appear to not be dose-related [8].

Other studies have shown that long-term neurological effects appear to persist such as Raynaud's phenomenon [11]. Additionally, there appears to be an effect on renal function in some patients followed long-term, although the clinical implications of these effects on renal function are unclear [12]. Finally, patients who receive platinum-based chemotherapy for testis cancer can have impairments in Leydig cell function in the long-term [13] (III/B).

The development of cisplatin-based chemotherapy has been life-saving for many thousands of patients with metastatic testis cancer. A patient with systemic metastatic disease requires cisplatin-based chemotherapy for cure and because the benefit is so great any morbidity is certainly acceptable. However, treating 50% of patients who in fact have no metastatic disease with chemotherapy exposes them to potential long-term side effects of the chemotherapy. This is especially pertinent since alternative methods of management (surveillance, nerve-sparing RPLND) exist, which do not subject patients with no metastatic disease to the potential side effects of chemotherapy.

Conclusions

Nerve-sparing RPLND is an effective single agent with low morbidity. Because removal of involved lymph nodes is curative at the 50%-75% level, nerve-sparing RPLND decreases the requirement for chemotherapy in the overall group of clinical stage I non-seminoma patients. Since the short-term chance for cure between the three methods of management (surveillance, nerve-sparing RPLND, and primary chemotherapy) is essentially the same, the choice of therapy in an individual patient is contingent upon local capabilities, patient desires, and availability of follow-up. Adequate informed consent is therefore essential in this group of patients.

Chapter 5

Recommendations	Evidence level

High risk

- High risk disease is denoted by embryonal carcinoma and vascular/ lymphatic invasion.   II/B

Chance for cure

- NS RPLND, surveillance and primary chemotherapy are curative at the 99% level.   III/B

Why nerve-sparing RPLND?

- Lymphatic metastasis may be cured merely by surgical excision of involved nodes.   III/B

Arguments against chemotherapy

- Chemotherapy is associated with long-term side effects.   III/B

References

1. Read G, Stenning SP, Cullen MH, Parkinson MC, Horwich A, Kaye SB, Cook PA. Medical Research Council Prospective study of surveillance for stage I testicular teratoma. *J Clinical Oncol* 1992; 10: 1762-68.

2. Albers P, Siener R, Kliesch S, Weissbach L, Krege S, Sparwasser C, Schulze H, Heidenreich A, deRiese W, Loy V, Bierhoff E, Wittekind C, Fimmers R, Hartmann M. Risk factors for relapse in clinical stage I nonseminomatous testicular germ cell tumors: results of the German Testicular Cancer Study Group trial. *J Clinical Oncol* 2003; 21: 1505-12.

3. Sweeney CJ, Hermans BP, Heilman DK, Foster RS, Donohue JP, Einhorn LH. Results and outcome of retroperitoneal lymph node dissection for clinical stage I embryonal carcinoma - predominant testis cancer. *J Clinical Oncol* 2000; 18: 358-62.

4. Bohlen D, Borner M, Sonntag RW, Fey MF, Studer UE. Long-term results following adjuvant chemotherapy in patients with clinical stage I testicular nonseminomatous malignant germ cell tumors with high risk factors. *J Urol* 1999; 161: 1148-52.

5. Baniel J, Foster RS, Rowland RG, *et al.* Complications of primary retroperitoneal lymph node dissection. *J Urol* 1994; 152: 424-7.

6. Lampe H, Horwich A, Norman A, Nicholls J, Dearnaley D. Fertility after chemotherapy for testicular germ cell cancers. *J Clinical Oncol* 1997; 15: 239-45.

7. Cullen MH Stenning SP, Parkinson MC, Fossa SD, Kaye SB, Horwich AH, Harland SJ, Williams MV, Jakes R. Short-course adjuvant chemotherapy in high risk stage I nonseminomatous germ cell tumors of the testis: A Medical Research Council Report. *J Clinical Oncol* 1996; 14: 1106-13.

8. Huddart RA, Norman A, Shahidi M, Horwich A, Coward D, Nicholls J, Dearnaley D. Cardiovascular disease as a long-term complication of treatment for testicular cancer. *J Clinical Oncol* 2003; 21: 1513-23.

9. Petersen PM, Hansen SW, Giwercman A, Rorth M, Skakkebaek, NE. Dose-dependent impairment of testicular function in patients treated with cisplatin-based chemotherapy for germ cell cancer. *Ann Oncol* 1994; 5: 355-8.

10. Meinardi MT, Gietema JA, Vander Graaf WTA, van Veldhuisen DJ, Runne MA, Sluiter WJ, deVries EGE, Willemse PBH, Mulder NH, vanderBerg MP, Schratfordt Koops H, Sleijfer DT. Cardiovascular morbidity in long-term survivors of metastatic testicular cancer. *J Clinical Oncol* 2000; 18: 1725-32.

11. Bokemeyer C, Berger CC, Kuczyk M, Schmoll HJ. Evaluation of long-term toxicity after chemotherapy for testicular cancer. *J Clinical Oncol* 1996; 14: 2923-32.

12. Fossa SD, Aass N, Winderen M, Bormer OP, Olsen DR. Long-term renal function after treatment for malignant germ cell tumours. *Ann Oncol* 2002; 13: 222-8.

13. Strumberg D, Brugge S, Korn MW, Koeppen S, Ranft J, Scheiber G, Reiners C, Mockel C, Seeber S, Scheulen ME. Evaluation of long-term toxicity in patients after cisplatin-based chemotherapy for nonsemimomatous testicular cancer. *Ann Oncol* 2002; 13: 229-36.

Chapter 6

Surgery versus chemotherapy for high risk NSGCT: why chemotherapy?

Kerry A Cheong BMBS FRACP
Clinical Research Fellow, Medical Oncology
Kathryn F Chrystal MB ChB FRACP
Clinical Research Fellow, Medical Oncology
Peter G Harper LRCP MRCS MB BS MRCP
Consultant Medical Oncologist

GUY'S HOSPITAL, LONDON, UK

Introduction

Testicular cancer is a disease predominantly of young men and its incidence has increased over the past 25 years. The introduction of platinum-based combination chemotherapy has transformed testicular cancer into a highly curable disease with overall survival rates over 90%. The proportion of non-seminomatous germ cell tumours (NSGCT) presenting as stage I has nearly doubled during this period, and now accounts for 50%-65% of presentations. Whilst in advanced stage disease chemotherapy remains the only curative therapy option, the therapeutic dilemma for the clinician in the management of early stage patients relates to the excellent outcome for all treatment options. Three management strategies can be followed:

- Close surveillance with chemotherapy at relapse.
- Risk adapted strategy - immediate chemotherapy for high risk and close surveillance for low risk.
- Retroperitoneal lymph node dissection (RPLND) with tailored chemotherapy according to "pathology" of the resected nodes.

The overall survival for all these strategies approaches 100%. It is imperative that the management choice be tailored to the individual patient, as the aim of all treatments is to maintain the excellent prognosis whilst minimising the immediate and long-term toxicities including psychological morbidity. This chapter will review the evidence for the role of primary chemotherapy in the management of high risk stage I non-seminomatous germ cell tumours.

Is adjuvant treatment necessary for clinical stage I NSGCT?

Stage I NSGCT is disease confined to the testis with no evidence of nodal spread. This can be classified as "clinical" stage I when based on nodal assessment by CT imaging following orchidectomy, or as "pathological" stage I based on RPLND.

Historically, treatment of the retroperitoneal lymph nodes with either surgery or radiotherapy provided the only option for improving cure rates in early stage disease given the predilection for recurrence in this region. With the introduction of effective chemotherapy in advanced disease, trials were instigated investigating the option of close surveillance with salvage chemotherapy at the time of disease progression, in an attempt to reduce the over-treatment and morbidity associated with retroperitoneal clearance. The largest prospective observational study by Read *et al* involving 396 patients, demonstrated a recurrence rate of 27% following inguinal orchidectomy, 80% of relapses were within the first 12 months, and the majority were salvaged with chemotherapy resulting in a five-year overall survival rate of 98% **(IIa/B)**. These results were confirmed in several other prospective observational studies [1-3] and in a recent systematic review [4]. Subsequent analysis of these trials has however, identified a "high risk" group, who have a relapse rate approaching 50% and may be more appropriately managed by primary chemotherapy. This group represents approximately 20%-30% of all clinical stage I presentations [5].

What defines high risk?

A systematic review of clinical stage I studies have confirmed the following factors as strongly predictive of recurrence: vascular invasion (venous or lymphatic), embryonal histology, high tumour proliferative activity (assessed by MIB-1 antibody positivity) and the size of tumour [4] **(Ia/A)**. These factors, when taken in conjunction with current clinical staging investigations (CXR, CT abdomen/pelvis and tumour markers), allow the identification of a group where the risk of recurrence is approximately 50%. The most recent predictive model incorporating three histological factors (vascular invasion, more than 70% MIB-1, and 50% or greater percentage of embryonal carcinoma) in clinical stage I disease results in a positive predictive value of 63.6% [6] **(IIa/B)**.

The predominant limitation of clinical staging revolves around its reliance on size as an indicator for tumour involvement. Sensitivity can be increased by reducing the size criteria but is done so at the loss of specificity [7] **(IIa/B)**. Current CT scanning understages up to 30% of patients who have occult metastasis in the retroperitoneum. Newer functional imaging such as FDG-PET reflecting the higher metabolic activity of tumour tissue may provide a better non-surgical method of staging. It has been successfully used in the treatment of advanced disease by the detection of residual or occult disease. Several small series in clinical stage I disease have been published [8-10]. These were not stratified by risk category. Lassen *et al* reported the largest involving 46 patients. In this study, the positive predictive value for PET was 100% and sensitivity, 70%. These results were superior to conventional staging and will need confirmation in a larger prospective study. Using this technology only 8% of patients would be over-treated [8]. The addition of FDG-PET to standard clinical staging may be one way to increase the identification of a "high risk" group and a large randomised prospective study using baseline PET results to determine treatment strategy is currently recruiting in the UK.

Adjuvant chemotherapy for high risk

Which chemotherapy?

The advent of curative platinum-based chemotherapy for advanced germ cell tumours has led to its application in an adjuvant setting. Three cycles of BEP (bleomycin, etoposide and cisplatin) is considered the combination of choice given its proven efficacy in the good prognostic advanced setting [11] **(Ib/A)**. Subsequently, the number of cycles used in the adjuvant setting has been between two and three. Cisplatin is the platinum of choice as studies substituting it for carboplatin have demonstrated inferior results [12] **(Ib/A)**. The advanced studies have also demonstrated that in patients with good prognostic metastatic disease, bleomycin can be omitted without loss of efficacy provided an additional cycle of EP is administered (etoposide 500mg/m^2) [13] **(Ib/A)**.

The efficacy of primary chemotherapy in high risk stage I NSGCT

The efficacy of primary chemotherapy in high risk clinical stage I NSGCT patients has been demonstrated in several studies with the outcomes of over 340 patients fully published and the results of a further 300 patients presented in abstract only (Table 1) [14-19]. The largest prospective study was by

Cullen *et al* in 1996 [14]. One hundred and fourteen men were given two cycles of BEP if they fulfilled the MRC high risk criteria established from the work by Read *et al*. Eligible men were required to have three of the following histological factors: venous invasion, lymphatic invasion, absence of yolk sac elements or presence of undifferentiated elements [5]. Ninety percent started within two months of surgery. At a median follow-up of four years, 97% remain relapse-free. Two relapses, seven and 18 months respectively, and two deaths (one disease-related and one treatment) have been reported. In addition,

there was one case of a second primary testicular tumour. Short-term toxicity was predominantly nausea and vomiting with 27% G3 emesis despite prophylactic anti-emetics. Haematological toxicity was mild with less than 5% G3 leucopenia on D22. These trials were performed prior to the introduction of the $5HT_3$ antagonists which are now the standard of care for highly emetogenic chemotherapy. These agents have dramatically improved the control of chemotherapy-induced nausea and vomiting. Sensory neuropathy was reported in 11%, and 8% developed tinnitus **(IIa/B)**.

Table 1. Chemotherapy trials in high risk stage I NSGCT.

Study	N	Risk factors	Regimen	PFS
Cullen *et al* [14] (1987-1994) (IIa/B)	114	MRC criteria*	BEP x2	Estimated 98% at 2 years
Pont *et al* [19] (1985-2003) (IIa/B)	74	VI	BEP x2	97% with median f/u 70 months
Studer *et al* [18] (1985-2000) (IIa/B)	59	VI or pT4 or EC	PVB x2 (20) BEP x2 (39)	96.6% with median f/u 93 months
Böhlen *et al* [16] (1985-1994) (IIa/B)	59	EC or VI or infiltration of tunica albuginea or absence of yolk sac elements	PVB x2 (20) BEP x2 (39)	98.3% with median f/u of 93 months
Schefer *et al* [17] (1994-1999) (IIa/B)	42	EC or VI or pT2	BEP x1	97.5% with median f/u of 32 months
Dearnaley *et al* [15] (1994-1996) (IIa/B)	115	VI	BOP x2	98.3% at 1 year

PFS=progression-free survival

BEP= bleomycin, etoposide, cisplatin

PVB=cisplatin, vinblastine, bleomycin

BOP=bleomycin, vincristine, cisplatin

VI=vascular invasion; EC=embryonal carcinoma

* 3 of the following needed: VI (venous or lymphatic) or undifferentiated elements or absence of yolk sac elements

Chapter 6

Long-term toxicities of chemotherapy

One of the important considerations in choosing the appropriate form of management for high risk clinical stage I NSGCT is the balance between maintaining overall survival and both acute and long-term toxicities, given the young age of presentation. The most important long-term toxicities in this patient group relate to fertility, pulmonary toxicity secondary to bleomycin, ototoxicity and secondary malignancies. Most data however, come from patients treated with advanced disease where cumulative doses are significantly higher and there is a greater tumour burden. Two fully published adjuvant studies had planned long-term toxicity assessments; however, the compliance in general was poor and the follow-up relatively brief (nine months and two years post-chemotherapy). Cullen *et al* found a significant but asymptomatic decrease in lung diffusing capacity with a mean change of 15% (p=0.002). No other significant impairments were found in fertility or hearing [14]. Pont *et al* assessed similar late toxicities but also included psychosocial morbidity and lipid profile. No significant impairments were noted. His data were updated in abstract form in 2003 with the median follow-up for high risk patients of 70 months (range 7-207 months) with no late sequelae recognised [19, 20].

Bleomycin pulmonary toxicity

Bleomycin pulmonary toxicity (BPT) is a potentially disabling and fatal complication of chemotherapy, predominantly consisting of pulmonary fibrosis. Cumulative dose (>450,000iu) and impaired renal clearance are the two risk factors with the strongest level of evidence. Bleomycin can be excluded or substituted from combination platinum therapy in good prognostic advanced germ cell tumours but at the price of an increased number of cycles (BEP x 3 = EP x 4) or with increased marrow suppression (VIP). Adjuvant chemotherapy would in general limit exposure to between 180,000iu and 270,000iu. A large review of 835 patients treated with BEP was recently published and the prevalence of BPT in stage I patients was 2.5% compared to an overall rate of 6.5% (III/B) [21]. It would appear that the likelihood of significant BPT with the administration of adjuvant chemotherapy is low.

Fertility

It is estimated that 22%-63% of men diagnosed with germ cell tumours will have suboptimal sperm counts [22]. For the majority of men this will recover; more than 80% of men treated with surveillance only (median follow-up of over ten years) will achieve fatherhood when wished for [23]. The evidence specific to primary chemotherapy in high risk NSGCT is limited. Cisplatin is the drug primarily responsible for sterilisation in the standard chemotherapy regimens associated with germ cell tumours. Previous work from men with stage II or III NSGCT has found that a cumulative cisplatin dose of >600mg/m^2 (six cycles of BEP) was associated with severe oligospermia or azoospermia [24] (III/B). Pont *et al* noted that fertility appeared to reduce with cisplatin doses >400mg/m^2 (four cycles of BEP) in patients treated with advanced disease chemotherapy protocols [25] (III/B). Cullen *et al*, who looked at trials of adjuvant therapy, scheduled fertility assessments, although only 16 of 119 were able to complete this adequately. No significant difference was found pre- and post-chemotherapy in these samples [14]. Bohlen *et al* sent follow-up questionnaires three years post-chemotherapy to their cohort of patients with reasonable compliance (83%). No impairment of fertility was found with respect to intended paternity. Twenty-seven of the 59 men volunteered a semen sample at a median of 90 months post-chemotherapy and only four had low sperm counts. All patients had been exposed to 240mg/m^2 of cisplatin [26]. Pont *et al* obtained semen samples from 18 of 44 men two years post-chemotherapy and found no significant difference between the samples of men post-chemotherapy and those treated with surveillance [20].

Cardiovascular morbidity

Recent work has suggested that there is an increased risk for cardiovascular complications for long-term survivors (over ten years) of advanced testicular cancer. In comparison to the population data, Meinardi *et al* noted the observed to expected ratio (O/E) of cardiovascular events was 7.1 (95% CI, 1.9-18.3) for patients treated with chemotherapy only. All patients were treated prior to 1987 and therefore are unlikely to include patients undergoing adjuvant chemotherapy [27] (III/B). The increase in cardiac events was accompanied by higher rates of cardiovascular risk factors, in particular higher blood pressure, and high cholesterol. This finding was confirmed by Huddart et al [28] when they found a two-fold higher risk of developing cardiovascular disease in those patients treated with chemotherapy alone in comparison to those with early stage disease treated with observation alone. A similar increased risk was seen for those treated with radiotherapy alone. This study did not however find any difference in cholesterol levels or mean blood pressure between the groups. This cohort of patients also had treatment between 1982 and 1992 **(III/B)**. The number of patients receiving adjuvant chemotherapy was not stated. Clinical trials using adjuvant chemotherapy were recruiting during this time period at this institution [28]. There is no evidence currently to suggest that those patients treated with adjuvant chemotherapy are at higher risk for cardiovascular morbidity but long-term follow-up studies are awaited with interest.

Renal toxicity

Cisplatin is well known to be associated with nephrotoxicity, in particular renal tubular damage. Fossa et al [29] **(III/B)** prospectively investigated the long-term glomerular filtration rate (GFR) in 85 patients with germ cell tumours. They observed a mean reduction in GFR of 14%, 12-17 years after cisplatin-based chemotherapy, when compared to the patients undergoing RPLND only. The impairment in renal function had occurred by three months post-chemotherapy and thereafter remained stable. GFR reduction was related to the cumulative dose of cisplatin. Petersen et al [30] **(III/B)** found similar reductions in GFR in the initial period following chemotherapy; however, in their series, renal function had recovered to within normal range by 10-15 years of follow-up. The clinical significance of these renal changes is uncertain, although it has been postulated this may be one of the factors contributing to a higher level of hypertension observed in this group.

Secondary malignancies

Travis et al, in their review of over 28,000 survivors of testicular cancer treated with chemotherapy or radiotherapy, noted that the number of secondary malignancies was 5% with an O/E ratio of 1.43. This included over 3300 men with more than 20 years of follow-up. There was an excess of acute lymphocytic leukaemia, acute myeloid leukaemia, Non-Hodgkins lymphoma, melanoma, and cancers of the stomach, colon, rectum, pancreas, prostate, kidney, bladder and thyroid. The review is hampered by the fact that the rate of secondary malignancies for those who were treated by surgery or observation only is not available [22] **(III/B)**. It is not inconceivable that this group of patients has a higher than normal baseline risk for malignancy due to genetic predisposition in comparison to the age-adjusted risk for the general population. It is also not stated how many of these men received adjuvant chemotherapy.

Radiotherapy alone was found to increase the risk of leukaemia three-fold. A similar level of risk was noted for exposure to a cumulative cisplatin dose >600mg (equivalent to three cycles of BEP) with the risk doubling again with doses over 1000mg (equivalent to five cycles of BEP) [31, 32]. Etoposide is a well recognised leukaemogenic agent with doses >2000mg (equivalent to three cycles of BEP) significantly associated with higher rates of leukaemia. Doses less than this were associated with a rate of 0.37% [33] **(III/B)**. It is not yet known what the rate of secondary malignancies will be with primary chemotherapy. The doses administered are in general lower than those discussed above. Mature data on efficacy is awaited for the newer regimens using fewer cycles or less leukaemogenic combinations [15, 17].

Other adjuvant therapeutic options for high risk stage I NSGCT

Surveillance

The crux of effective surveillance strategies is compliance - requiring both motivated patients and staff. The range of compliance in published audits varies between 10%-65% with drop-out increasing with time post-orchidectomy. Nicolai et al [34] **(III/B)** noted that non-compliance resulted in a 30% increase in the mean time to follow-up in comparison to the suggested "best practice" follow-up protocols. Late presentation of advanced disease and subsequent inability to salvage is the principle concern with surveillance strategies. Only one audit suggested a poorer prognosis for those patients who were non-compliant - 20% of the relapsed but non-compliant group were not salvageable but the non-compliant subset consisted only of 29 patients. One of the postulated reasons for non-compliance is psychological morbidity associated with such intensive follow-up. This is perhaps one of the strongest arguments encountered for primary chemotherapy in high risk stage I disease. Assessment of this aspect of therapy was specifically addressed in only one study published so far. Pont *et al* did not demonstrate any significant difference between those men undergoing adjuvant chemotherapy compared to surveillance. Their quality of life (QoL) data suffered from a lower compliance rate in comparison to most QoL studies (16/25 returned compared with 22/27 in the adjuvant group) and additionally, a validated instrument was not administered [20]. Formal QoL assessments are now routinely administered in the newer studies but their results are awaited.

Retroperitoneal lymph node dissection

The disease-free recurrence rate achieved with primary chemotherapy compares favourably with the outcomes seen with RPLND. These are highly dependent on the expertise of the surgeon. The most common long-term morbidity remains ejaculatory dysfunction (1%-15% depending on technique and centre) and small bowel obstruction (1%). The Indiana group, which has the most extensive surgical experience, reports a recurrence rate post-RPLND of 11%; however, patients with pathological stage II disease (following positive histology at RPLND) in this centre will generally receive two cycles of adjuvant chemotherapy, i.e. surgery plus chemotherapy. The likelihood of recurrence in this group is dependent on the number of positive lymph nodes: up to 80%-85% of men will remain disease-free post-RPLND if less than three lymph nodes are involved, all nodes are less than 2cm in size and there is no extranodal extension on histological review [35] **(IIa/B)**.

Conclusions

Three treatment options are available for the high risk clinical stage I patient, all of which potentially confer equivalent long-term outcomes. No studies have directly compared these strategies.

Primary chemotherapy

If all patients are treated with 2-3 cycles of chemotherapy, then 50% of patients are potentially receiving unnecessary chemotherapy, with the associated risks of toxicity. The majority of patients however, will be cured up-front with only 3% of patients requiring further chemotherapy for relapse.

Adjuvant chemotherapy for high risk NSGCT is an effective means of reducing the risk of recurrence, subsequent additional surgery and prolonged chemotherapy, but conveys no survival advantage over other therapeutic options. Toxicities are acceptable; however, the evidence for long-term toxicity is limited. It should be considered on an individual basis but especially for those patients in whom compliance may be an issue or if they have significant anxiety associated with a surveillance strategy. Improved non-invasive imaging techniques in addition to histological factors will aid in identifying the high risk group.

Retroperitoneal lymph node dissection

All patients would be operated on, thus exposing all to the potential complications of surgery. Accurate assessment of the nodes will be obtained and historical studies suggest that 20%-30% of clinical stage I patients will be pathological stage II after RPLND [36]. Currently, these patients (20%) receive adjuvant chemotherapy. Historical studies also demonstrate that 10%-17% of pathological stage I patients will relapse outside of the retroperitoneum despite surgery, and will require treatment with an advanced disease protocol. In addition, a small number of patients will not be salvaged with the current advanced disease protocol. In field relapse is often dependent on the expertise of the surgeon and recurrence rates vary between 1%-10% [36, 37]. These patients may require further surgery.

Surveillance and treatment on relapse

This avoids unnecessary chemotherapy or surgery in 50% of patients. The remainder though will be subjected to treatment using an advanced disease protocol at relapse which is associated with a greater number of cycles and subsequent exposure to higher cumulative doses of chemotherapy. In addition, 5%-15% of patients will require surgery as part of salvage therapy. A small number of patients will not be salvaged with current treatments. Surveillance relies on excellent compliance from both patient and clinician.

Who should definitely receive primary chemotherapy?

Analysis of those patients who relapse post-RPLND have identified a group of patients who would benefit from primary chemotherapy in preference to RPLND. This group has persistently elevated markers post-orchidectomy and this was found to be an independent predictor of relapse with a relative risk of 8.0 [38-40]. It is highly likely that this group has micrometastases outside of the retroperitoneal lymph nodes **(III/B)**.

Future directions

Decreasing the number of cycles of chemotherapy, and lessening its toxicity, particularly fertility and secondary tumours, are important ways forward. Preliminary data on the efficacy of one cycle of adjuvant chemotherapy have been published and mature data are awaited with interest [17, 41]. Early results are also available for "etoposide-free" regimens, acknowledging that etoposide is the primary agent responsible for the development of leukaemia [15, 41]. Taxanes are now being routinely used in the advanced setting but have so far not been studied in the adjuvant setting. The difficulty with the introduction of newer agents into primary chemotherapy for high risk clinical stage I NSGCT is its excellent current prognosis. Any small advantage will take large trials to detect this, probably involving 1000 patients. Studies comparing directly RPLND with adjuvant chemotherapy are currently underway and results are awaited. Quality of life assessment has been incorporated into many of these newer studies and this information will be useful to help guide future treatment decisions, given the equivalence of them all in terms of long-term outcome. The influence of growth factors eg. G-CSF in minimising haematological toxicity associated with adjuvant chemotherapy has yet to be fully explored. It is well recognised that maintenance of dose intensity in the advanced setting has led to gains in survival and these growth factors have been important in minimising the risks of infection with prolonged neutropenia.

Chapter 6

Chapter 6

Recommendations	Evidence level

Does chemotherapy prevent recurrence?

- Yes, adjuvant chemotherapy reduces the risk of recurrence in high risk patients. — IIa/B

Does adjuvant chemotherapy confer a survival advantage?

- No, compared to close surveillance and salvage chemotherapy on relapse, survival outcomes are equivalent. — IIa/B

How many cycles of chemotherapy are required for stage I high risk NSGCT?

- Two cycles of BEP is the current standard of care. Data are awaited for one cycle or "etoposide-free" regimens. — IIa/B

Does adjuvant chemotherapy result in significant long-term toxicity?

- There is no evidence of impaired fertility or hearing loss with adjuvant chemotherapy. — IIa/B
- Long-term data in patients receiving chemotherapy for advanced disease (≥ 3 cycles) suggest increased cardiovascular morbidity and secondary malignancies. No long-term data are available for adjuvant chemotherapy.

References

1. Gels ME, Hoekstra HJ, Sleijfer DT, Marrink J, de Bruijn HW, Molenaar WM, et al. Detection of recurrence in patients with clinical stage I nonseminomatous testicular germ cell tumors and consequences for further follow-up: a single-center 10-year experience. J Clin Oncol 1995; 13(5): 1188-94.

2. Sogani PC, Perrotti M, Herr HW, Fair WR, Thaler HT, Bosl G. Clinical stage I testis cancer: long-term outcome of patients on surveillance. J Urol 1998; 159(3): 855-8.

3. Sturgeon JF, Jewett MA, Alison RE, Gospodarowicz MK, Blend R, Herman S, et al. Surveillance after orchidectomy for patients with clinical stage I nonseminomatous testis tumors. J Clin Oncol 1992; 10(4): 564-8.

4. Vergouwe Y, Steyerberg EW, Eijkemans MJ, Albers P, Habbema JD. Predictors of occult metastasis in clinical stage I nonseminoma: a systematic review. J Clin Oncol 2003; 21(22): 4092-9.

5. Read G, Stenning SP, Cullen MH, Parkinson MC, Horwich A, Kaye SB, et al. Medical Research Council prospective study of surveillance for stage I testicular teratoma. Medical Research Council Testicular Tumors Working Party. J Clin Oncol 1992; 10(11): 1762-8.

6. Albers P, Siener R, Kliesch S, Weissbach L, Krege S, Sparwasser C, et al. Risk factors for relapse in clinical stage I nonseminomatous testicular germ cell tumors: results of the German Testicular Cancer Study Group Trial. J Clin Oncol 2003; 21(8): 1505-12.

7. Leibovitch L, Foster RS, Kopecky KK, Donohue JP. Improved accuracy of computerized tomography-based clinical staging in low stage nonseminomatous germ cell cancer using size criteria of retroperitoneal lymph nodes. J Urol 1995; 154(5): 1759-63.

8. Lassen U, Daugaard G, Eigtved A, Hojgaard L, Damgaard K, Rorth M. Whole-body FDG-PET in patients with stage I non-seminomatous germ cell tumours. Eur J Nucl Med Mol Imaging 2003; 30(3): 396-402.

9. Albers P, Bender H, Yilmaz H, Schoeneich G, Biersack HJ, Mueller SC. Positron emission tomography in the clinical staging of patients with Stage I and II testicular germ cell tumors. Urology 1999; 53(4): 808-11.

10. Hain SF, O'Doherty MJ, Timothy AR, Leslie MD, Partridge SE, Huddart RA. Fluorodeoxyglucose PET in the initial staging of germ cell tumours. Eur J Nucl Med 2000; 27(5): 590-4.

11. de Wit R, Roberts JT, Wilkinson PM, de Mulder PH, Mead GM, Fossa SD, et al. Equivalence of three or four cycles of bleomycin, etoposide, and cisplatin chemotherapy and of a

3- or 5-day schedule in good-prognosis germ cell cancer: a randomized study of the European Organization for Research and Treatment of Cancer Genitourinary Tract Cancer Cooperative Group and the Medical Research Council. *J Clin Oncol* 2001; 19(6): 1629-40.

12. Bajorin DF, Sarosdy MF, Pfister DG, Mazumdar M, Motzer RJ, Scher HI, *et al.* Randomized trial of etoposide and cisplatin versus etoposide and carboplatin in patients with good-risk germ cell tumors: a multiinstitutional study. *J Clin Oncol* 1993; 11(4): 598-606.

13. Toner GC, Stockler MR, Boyer MJ, Jones M, Thomson DB, Harvey VJ, *et al.* Comparison of two standard chemotherapy regimens for good-prognosis germ-cell tumours: a randomised trial. Australian and New Zealand Germ Cell Trial Group. *Lancet* 2001; 357(9258): 739-45.

14. Cullen MH, Stenning SP, Parkinson MC, Fossa SD, Kaye SB, Horwich AH, *et al.* Short-course adjuvant chemotherapy in high-risk stage I nonseminomatous germ cell tumors of the testis: a Medical Research Council report. *J Clin Oncol* 1996; 14(4): 1106-13.

15. Dearnaley DP, Fossa SD, Kaye SB, Harland SJ, Roberts JT, Sokal M, *et al.* Adjuvant bleomycin, vincristine and cisplatin (BOP) for high risk clinical stage I (HRCS1) non-seminomatous germ cell tumours (NSGCT) - a Medical Research Council (MRC) pilot study. In: *Proc Soc Clin Oncol* 1998; 309a, abst 1189.

16. Bohlen D, Borner M, Sonntag RW, Fey MF, Studer UE. Long-term results following adjuvant chemotherapy in patients with clinical stage I testicular nonseminomatous malignant germ cell tumors with high risk factors. *J Urol* 1999; 161(4): 1148-52.

17. Schefer H, Mattmann S, Borner M, Morant R, Studer UE, Nandedkar M, *et al.* Single course of adjuvant bleomycin, etoposide and cisplatin (BEP) for high risk stage I non-seminomatous germ cell tumours (NSGCT). In: *Proc Soc Clin Oncol* 2003; Chicago, 2003: p.abst 1339.

18. Studer UE, Burkhard FC, Sonntag RW. Risk adapted management with adjuvant chemotherapy in patients with high risk clinical stage I nonseminomatous germ cell tumor. *J Urol* 2000; 163(6): 1785-7.

19. Pont J, De Santis M, Albrecht W, Scholtz M, Hoetl W. Risk adapted management for clinical stage I nonseminomatous germ cell cancer of the testis (NSGCT I) by regarding vascular invasion (VI): a 17-year experience from the Vienna Testicular Tumour Study Group. In: *Proc Am Soc Clin Oncol* 2003; Chicago, 2003: 388, abst 1558.

20. Pont J, Albrecht W, Postner G, Sellner F, Angel K, Holtl W. Adjuvant chemotherapy for high-risk clinical stage I nonseminomatous testicular germ cell cancer: long-term results of a prospective trial. *J Clin Oncol* 1996; 14(2): 441-8.

21. O'Sullivan JM, Huddart RA, Norman AR, Nicholls J, Dearnaley DP, Horwich A. Predicting the risk of bleomycin lung toxicity in patients with germ-cell tumours. *Ann Oncol* 2003; 14(1): 91-6.

22. Gaffan J, Holden L, Newlands ES, Short D, Fuller S, Begent RH, *et al.* Infertility rates following POMB/ACE chemotherapy for male and female germ cell tumours - a retrospective long-term follow-up study. *Br J Cancer* 2003; 89(10): 1849-54.

23. Herr HW, Bar-Chama N, O'Sullivan M, Sogani PC. Paternity in men with stage I testis tumors on surveillance. *J Clin Oncol* 1998; 16(2): 733-4.

24. Petersen PM, Hansen SW, Giwercman A, Rorth M, Skakkebaek NE. Dose-dependent impairment of testicular function in patients treated with cisplatin-based chemotherapy for germ cell cancer. *Ann Oncol* 1994; 5(4): 355-8.

25. DeSantis M, Albrecht W, Holtl W, Pont J. Impact of cytotoxic treatment on long-term fertility in patients with germ-cell cancer. *Int J Cancer* 1999; 83(6): 864-5.

26. Bohlen D, Burkhard FC, Mills R, Sonntag RW, Studer UE. Fertility and sexual function following orchiectomy and 2 cycles of chemotherapy for stage I high risk nonseminomatous germ cell cancer. *J Urol* 2001; 165(2): 441-4.

27. Meinardi MT, Gietema JA, van der Graaf WT, van Veldhuisen DJ, Runne MA, Sluiter WJ, *et al.* Cardiovascular morbidity in long-term survivors of metastatic testicular cancer. *J Clin Oncol* 2000; 18(8): 1725-32.

28. Huddart RA, Norman A, Shahidi M, Horwich A, Coward D, Nicholls J, *et al.* Cardiovascular disease as a long-term complication of treatment for testicular cancer. *J Clin Oncol* 2003; 21(8): 1513-23.

29. Fossa SD, Aass N, Winderen M, Bormer OP, Olsen DR. Long-term renal function after treatment for malignant germ-cell tumours. *Ann Oncol* 2002; 13(2): 222-8.

30. Petersen PM, Hansen SW. The course of long-term toxicity in patients treated with cisplatin-based chemotherapy for non-seminomatous germ-cell cancer. *Ann Oncol* 1999; 10(12): 1475-83.

31. Travis LB, Curtis RE, Storm H, Hall P, Holowaty E, Van Leeuwen FE, *et al.* Risk of second malignant neoplasms among long-term survivors of testicular cancer. *J Natl Cancer Inst* 1997; 89(19): 1429-39.

32. Travis LB, Andersson M, Gospodarowicz M, van Leeuwen FE, Bergfeldt K, Lynch CF, *et al.* Treatment-associated leukemia following testicular cancer. *J Natl Cancer Inst* 2000; 92(14): 1165-71.

33. Nichols CR, Breeden ES, Loehrer PJ, Williams SD, Einhorn LH. Secondary leukemia associated with a conventional dose of etoposide: review of serial germ cell tumor protocols. *J Natl Cancer Inst* 1993; 85(1): 36-40.

34. Nicolai N, Pizzocaro G. A surveillance study of clinical stage I nonseminomatous germ cell tumors of the testis: 10-year follow-up. *J Urol* 1995; 154(3): 1045-9.

35. Rabbani F, Sheinfeld J, Farivar-Mohseni H, Leon A, Rentzepis MJ, Reuter VE, *et al.* Low-volume nodal metastases detected at retroperitoneal lymphadenectomy for testicular cancer: pattern and prognostic factors for relapse. *J Clin Oncol* 2001; 19(7): 2020-5.

36. Sweeney CJ, Hermans BP, Heilman DK, Foster RS, Donohue JP, Einhorn LH. Results and outcome of retroperitoneal lymph node dissection for clinical stage I embryonal carcinoma-predominant testis cancer. *J Clin Oncol* 2000; 18(2): 358-62.

37. Heidenreich A, Albers P, Hartmann M, Kliesch S, Kohrmann KU, Krege S, *et al.* Complications of primary nerve-sparing retroperitoneal lymph node dissection for clinical stage I nonseminomatous germ cell tumors of the testis: experience

of the German Testicular Cancer Study Group. *J Urol* 2003;
169(5): 1710-4.

38. Culine S, Theodore C, Terrier-Lacombe MJ, Droz JP. Primary
chemotherapy in patients with nonseminomatous germ cell
tumors of the testis and biological disease only after
orchiectomy. *J Urol* 1996; 155(4): 1296-8.

39. Davis BE, Herr HW, Fair WR, Bosl GJ. The management of
patients with nonseminomatous germ cell tumors of the testis
with serologic disease only after orchiectomy. *J Urol* 1994;
152(1): 111-3; discussion 114.

40. Saxman SB, Nichols CR, Foster RS, Messemer JE, Donohue
JP, Einhorn LH. The management of patients with clinical
stage I nonseminomatous testicular tumors and persistently
elevated serologic markers. *J Urol* 1996; 155(2): 587-9.

41. Klepp O, Dahl O, Cavallin-Stahl E, Stierner U, Cohn
Cedermark G, Wist E, *et al*. Risk-adapted, brief adjuvant
chemotherapy in clinical stage I (CS1) nonseminomatous
germ cell testicular cancer (NSHCT). In: *Proc Soc Clin Oncol*
2003; Chicago, 2003: 399, abst 1604.

Chapter 6

Chapter 7

Timing of orchidopexy for undescended testes

Stephen J Griffin MMedSc FRCS Ed
Specialist Registrar, Urology

EDITH CAVELL HOSPITAL, PETERBOROUGH, UK

Introduction

An undescended testis (UDT) is defined as the arrest of the testicle in its normal pathway of descent from the germinal ridge on the posterior abdominal wall to the scrotum. Deviation from this normal course is called an ectopic testis. Both situations lead to an absent scrotal testis, termed cryptorchidism (*kryptos*, meaning hidden and *orchis* representing testicle). Testicular descent has taxed the minds of surgeons since the time of Hunter in the 18th century [1]. Hunter questioned whether the testes did not descend because of dysgenesis or whether failure to descend induced dysgenesis [2]. Cooper discovered that very young children with cryptorchid testes can have histologically normal testes. She observed that the degree of dysgenesis appears related to the manner of proximal arrest of descent [3]. Backhouse proposed that testicular maldescent might result from hormonal failure; abnormal levels of testosterone, dihydro-testosterone or Mullerian Inhibiting Substance may affect descent. Furthermore, hormonal failure may lead to a shortened testicular artery or vas deferens further hampering descent mechanically [4].

UDT is one of the commonest congenital abnormalities and the incidence is rising. Scorer, in the 1950s, assessed approximately 3600 babies classifying cryptorchidism by measurement [5]. A testis was considered cryptorchid if the centre was less than 4cm below the pubic tubercle (2.5cm at birth examination for babies <2500g). Approximately 4% of male infants had cryptorchidism at birth. This fell to 0.96% and 0.8% at three and 12 months respectively. The John Radcliffe Hospital Cryptorchidism Study Group prospectively assessed almost 7500 male births in the mid 1980s for UDT [6]. Using the same examination techniques as Scorer, UDT rates at birth and three months increased to 5.4% and 1.85% respectively. Approximately 2% had bilateral cryptorchidism at birth falling to nearly 1% at three months. Factors which predicted normal testicular descent at three months were low birth weight, bilateral cryptorchidism and normal scrotal size.

The incidence of UDT further rises to 4%-6% at age 5-11 years. High rates of spontaneous descent at puberty lead to a reduction to 1% again at adolescence [7]. The recently described *acquired* form of UDT [8] probably accounts for the higher orchidopexy rates later in childhood in most countries.

UDT is associated with inguinal hernia [9] and altered body image in childhood [10] and infertility [11] and testicular cancer later in life [12, 13].

Orchidopexy is one of the most common surgical procedures in childhood and forms the corner stone for management of UDT. The aim of the procedure is to improve cosmesis, repair a concomitant hernia or patent processus vaginalis (56%-100% incidence with congenital UDT [9, 14]), optimise later fertility, allow testicular examination and possibly decrease testicular cancer risk. There has been considerable debate in the literature over the years as to the best time to perform orchidopexy. Furthermore, it has been questioned whether orchidopexy is always required for treatment of acquired UDT. This chapter will explore the evidence base for current practice and examine whether the time at which orchidopexy is performed impacts upon the infertility level, testicular cancer rates, or the psychological distress associated with UDT. It will also explore the evidence for treatment of acquired UDT.

Fertility

It is well known that testes which remain undescended through puberty will be sterile later in life. Using 20 million sperm/ml as a definition of fertility, analysis of various series by Kogan [15] calculated mean fertility rates of 51.5% and 28.5% for unilateral and bilateral UDT respectively **(III/B)**.

A review of 27 papers that considered adult fertility in terms of sperm density revealed that, after treatment, 57% of patients with unilateral cryptorchidism and 25% of patients with bilateral cryptorchidism had sperm densities greater than 20 million/ml [16] **(III/B)**. A more recent study of paternity revealed no significant difference between unilateral UDT paternity rates versus controls (75% and 76% respectively) [17], although only 53% of those with bilateral UDT had fathered a child **(IIa/B)**. However, paternity in this study was self-reported. Such measurements are fraught with obvious problems and may tend to overestimate the true incidence of fertility. Furthermore, iatrogenic injury causing testicular atrophy (5% of cases [18]) may make future assessment of fertility inaccurate.

In 1960, Charny [18] stated that testicular biopsy in a large number of testes brought into the scrotum failed to reveal a single instance of normal spermatogenesis. Operative techniques (at that time) yielded better cosmetic than functional results and it was recommended that boys with asymptomatic UDT and no clinically recognised hernia should be spared the hazard and inconvenience of orchidopexy! However, this statement was made at a time when orchidopexy was not being performed on boys at really young ages. Does this then impact upon fertility rates?

As early as 1929 histological evidence revealed that undescended testicles expressed morphological changes as early as the third year of life [3]. Cooper compared histological findings in retained and scrotal testes of similar age. She noted by age 2½ years that the undescended testes had decreased numbers of seminiferous tubules and increased interstitial stroma. Furthermore, tubular cells were normal in appearance but decreased in number **(III/B)**. This work went largely unheeded until work in the 1970s and 1980s. By using spermatogonia count, in addition to qualitative examination of the ultra-structure of the interstitial tissue, in the assessment of 578 malpositioned testes, Mengel and colleagues [19] showed in almost all cases that the undescended testes had no histomorphological changes during the first two years of life. The mean values of spermatogonia counts were within normal range initially, but decreased significantly after the second year **(IIb/B)**.

Hedinger evaluated over 600 testicular biopsies from 450 boys with unilateral or bilateral cryptorchidism between age two months and ten years [20]. Mean spermatogonia counts were the same in the normally descended testes and undescended testes during the first year of life. A difference between the two groups was observed in the second and third years, and thereafter, significantly lower counts were found in the cryptorchid group and counts remained low until puberty **(IIb/B)**.

Electron microscopic studies comparing undescended testes with normal controls [21] have revealed no morphological alterations in spermatogonia in the first year of life, but increased collagen in the peritubular tissue of the undescended testicles from the second year and thickening of the tunica propria from the third year. These changes become more pronounced with age. Furthermore, cryptorchid testes were found to have underdeveloped leydig cells from early in life **(IIb/B)**.

A more recent study described interstitial fibrosis with increased collagen deposition as the most clearly defined morphological finding in the cryptorchid testes [22]. This finding was evident before age one and progressed with time **(III/B)**.

Histological evidence has led some authors [19-22] to recommend orchidopexy for UDT before age two **(IIb/B)**. However, only two studies [19,20] have large numbers of subjects and neither use completely normal testes as controls.

Initial clinical evidence that orchidopexy at a really young age may be beneficial was provided by Ludwig and Potempa [23]. In 71 patients, who underwent orchidopexy for unilateral UDT between the first and 13th years, fertility rate correlated directly with earlier date of operation **(III/B)**. Approximately 90% of those undergoing operation from 0-2 years were fertile. This dropped to under 60% when the operation was performed between the third and fourth years and to 25% between the ninth and 12th years.

Hedinger [20] assessed descended testes from subjects with unilateral UDT as controls. Although the spermatogonia count in these testicles is better than the undescended testes, they have lower mean values than completely normal controls [19]. Less than ten subjects were included in each of the other studies [21, 22] and controls were only used in one [21]. No comment was made as to whether these were truly normal or descended testes in subjects with UDT. Even so, one could imagine impossible difficulties obtaining approval and consent for testicular biopsy in truly normal controls for such a study.

Furthermore, early orchidopexy is safe [24]. Evaluation of 77 patients between 2-46 months old undergoing orchidopexy for UDT revealed an overall complication rate of less than 4% (3/77). Only one patient, aged 28 months, had testicular atrophy (1.3%). Another study quotes a 5% testicular atrophy rate in each of two groups undergoing orchidopexy before and after their second birthday [18].

Chilvers and colleagues' review [16] of adult fertility following diagnosis and treatment of UDT concluded that only treatment of bilateral UDT improves fertility rates. Prior to treatment, all bilateral cryptorchids were azoospermic or oligospermic. Post-treatment 25% of this group had sperm counts greater than 20 million/ml. In the unilateral group, 56% had normal sperm counts before treatment compared to 57% after treatment. They further concluded that age at operation has no effect on subsequent fertility. However, in the papers reviewed, orchidopexy was generally performed between 4-14 years. Furthermore, only seven of the 27 papers provided information on orchidopexy timing.

Semen analysis of 142 men over 18 years, who underwent orchidopexy for UDT at a single centre between 7-13½ years of age, revealed 74% had normal sperm density and therefore had a reasonable chance of fertility [25]. The main risk factors for impaired fertility in this study were initial high position of the testicle or bilateral UDT, not timing of orchidopexy **(III/B)**. However, only 43% (142/329) of the group undergoing late orchidopexy, provided semen for analysis. Furthermore, no comparison was made to the other 182 patients who presumably had earlier orchidopexy over the study period (511 patients in total).

A recent comparison of paternity rates in men with a history of unilateral UDT and controls concluded there was no correlation between age at orchidopexy and paternity [17] **(IIa/B)**. However, only 8.6% (18/209), attempting paternity, had their orchidopexy under two years of age.

More recently, an attempt was made to correlate tubular diameter and tubular fertility index to age at orchidopexy in testicular biopsy specimens, from a large number of cryptorchid patients who had undergone orchidopexy [14]. Although no statistical relationship between timing of orchidopexy and tubular fertility index or tubular diameter were found, the most normal values were those obtained from children in the first year of life **(III/B)**. The authors therefore recommended that orchidopexy should be undertaken for UDT as soon as possible before two years of age **(III/B)**.

The fact that the clinical evidence is not as strong as the histological evidence for early orchidopexy, at this point in time, is hardly surprising as this policy was deemed new in the 1980s [26]. Evaluation has to wait for the boys, who were operated on before their second birthday, to be able to provide semen specimens and father children.

Testicular cancer

The increased risk of testicular cancer with cryptorchidism has been established for more than 140 years [12]. The aetiology of testicular malignancy in cryptorchidism has not been elucidated. Various theories have been proposed including trauma, the effect of the altered environment on developing seminiferous tubules, temperature elevation, germinal atrophy, hormonal imbalance and inherent germ cell defect [27] **(IV/C)**. The relative risk of testicular cancer associated with UDT was 20-46 in earlier series [28] **(III/B)**. Approximately 15% of the testes were located intra-abdominally, but these accounted for nearly 50% of the malignancies. This represents a six-fold increase in risk in intra-abdominal testes compared to low-lying cryptorchid testes. More recent case-control series report a relative risk of 5-10 [12, 16, 29] **(III/B)**. Approximately 10% of patients with testicular cancer have a history of cryptorchidism [16].

In a retrospective population-based case-control study, Forman and colleagues [13] looked at the association between UDT and testicular cancer. They compared 794 men with testicular germ cell tumours diagnosed over a three-year period with age-matched controls. Diagnosis of UDT was confirmed by review of general practitioners' notes. This revealed a relative risk of 3.82 **(III/B)**. The authors suggest two reasons for the lower risk compared to that found in other studies: seeking verification of UDT diagnosis from general practitioners' notes and the possibility of increasing incidence of UDT.

Furthermore, results suggested that men who had unilateral UDT corrected before age ten were no longer at increased risk of testicular cancer. As only one orchidopexy was performed before age five, this study did not lend support for orchidopexy at particularly young ages, but the authors suggested the trend to reduce age at orchidopexy should be encouraged.

Martin and colleagues [28] have reported 220 cases of germinal cell tumours that occurred after orchidopexy. Ninety-seven cases were described in enough detail to conclude that the testicle remained permanently in the scrotum. Mean time between orchidopexy and tumour diagnosis was ten years. Only six of the 97 had their orchidopexy performed before age ten **(III/B)**. This supports the notion that earlier orchidopexy may decrease the subsequent risk of testicular cancer. Martin further states that orchidopexy in the second year may allow full maturation of the testicle limiting the later development of testicular malignancy **(IV/C)**.

A retrospective review of 1075 boys with cryptorchidism has shown that the relative risk of testicular cancer falls significantly 15 years after orchidopexy [12]. However, in this study, the age at orchidopexy had no effect on testicular cancer risk **(III/B)**. Pike and colleagues [30] reviewed a cohort of 58 patients from a single centre with testicular cancer who had orchidopexy or orchidectomy previously for UDT. They compared the age at orchidopexy in this group of patients with the expected age distribution for orchidopexy in all patients with UDT and concluded that age at orchidopexy had no effect on testicular cancer risk **(III/B)**. However, only four of the 57 patients evaluated had their orchidopexy before age five. Furthermore, they were unable to ascertain the initial testicular position of the testicle prior to orchidopexy as operative notes had been destroyed in all except five cases.

As adverse histological changes are seen in cryptorchid testes at age two, it may be that orchidopexy done at this age may reduce risk. However, data are lacking [12] **(IV/C)**. Some studies suggest that bilateral UDT confers increased risk [12, 31] **(III/B)**. This would fit with the theory that an abnormal hormonal milieu from the hypothalamic-pituitary-gonadal axis leads to compromised interstitial and germinal cell development causing maldescent and variable tubular dysgenesis [27].

Although evidence suggests earlier orchidopexy (less than ten years old) may limit the development of testicular cancer [13, 28], there is currently no evidence that orchidopexy under two years old further limits testicular cancer development. However, men who initially had their orchidopexy for UDT before their second birthday will only now be coming of age to develop testicular cancer.

Acquired UDT

In acquired UDT, a previously documented scrotal testis can no longer be manipulated into a stable position in the scrotum with further traction on the cord being painful [7] **(III/B)**. This condition is two to three times more common than congenital UDT. It may be primary ("ascending testis") or secondary following ipsilateral groin surgery ("trapped testis").

A retrospective review of over 600 children who underwent nearly 750 groin explorations for inguinal hernia revealed the incidence of secondary acquired UDT was 1.3% under five years old and 0.75% for those above age five years [32] **(III/B)**. A series of more than 100 boys undergoing orchidopexy revealed congenital UDT was always associated with a complete hernial sac whereas approximately 70% of those recorded as having a descended testis neonatally (primary acquired UDT) did not have an associated hernia [9] **(III/B)** suggesting an alternative aetiological process in this condition. Conversely, two smaller series found an associated patent processus vaginalis in the majority of boys with this condition [33,34] **(III/B)**. Preliminary results of an ongoing prospective study observing the natural course of acquired UDT show that approximately 80% of primary acquired UDT will descend spontaneously at puberty with appropriate testicular volumes for age [7] **(III/B)**.

The aetiology of primary acquired UDT is unknown. Selected series suggest it is due to partial absorption of a patent processus vaginalis [33, 34] **(IV/C)**. This is not supported by findings from a larger study where the majority of boys did not have an associated hernial sac [9]. Although primary acquired UDT is usually treated with orchidopexy for cosmesis or at parental request [8] **(IV/C)**, watchful waiting until puberty is reasonable [7] **(III/B)**. To date, there is no evidence that earlier operation prevents impaired spermatogenesis in this group. Indeed, the risk of testicular malignancy and infertility could differ in acquired UDT compared to those with congenital UDT [9] **(IV/C)**.

Secondary acquired UDT has various postulated causes: retractile testes getting trapped in the scar tissue at the site of hernia repair or groin exploration, suturing the testicle or cord whilst closing the external oblique aponeurosis or failure to replace the testis in the scrotum if it is pulled up into the wound during groin exploration [32] **(IV/C)**. Meticulous technique and formal orchidopexy or cremasteric myotomy in those with retractile testes (more common under five years old) noted prior to groin exploration may limit this occurrence [35]. When it occurs, it is best treated with orchidopexy [8] **(IV/C)**.

Psychological factors

As evidence suggests germ cell numbers decrease with delayed orchidopexy, and since orchidopexy performed by paediatric sub-specialists confers no greater risk to young children, the American Academy of Paediatrics recommend operation soon after age one [10]. Furthermore, from a psychological standpoint, they argue that it is better to have surgery before age two **(IV/C)**. From six weeks to 15 months of age, surgery seems to cause relatively less psychological distress if parental separation is limited. In addition, children under two years of age require relatively little cognitive preparation for surgery.

Recommendations	Evidence level
◆ The incidence of UDT is approximately 1% at age one.	III/B
◆ After treatment, approximately 60% of patients with unilateral cryptorchidism, and 25% of patients with bilateral cryptorchidism, have normal sperm densities.	III/B
◆ Unilateral cryptorchids have near normal paternity rates, but bilateral rates are reduced.	IIa/B
◆ Histological evidence suggests orchidopexy for UDT should be performed between ages 1-2 years to optimise later fertility.	IIb/B
◆ To date, the *clinical* evidence to support early orchidopexy to maximise fertility is not as strong. This may come with prospective analysis of semen samples and paternity rates of large numbers of males who have undergone orchidopexy for UDT before their second birthday.	
◆ Relative risk of testicular cancer with UDT is 4-10.	III/B
◆ Intra-abdominal testes and bilateral cryptorchidism confer increased risk of testicular cancer.	III/B
◆ There is conflicting epidemiological evidence that orchidopexy before age ten might decrease the risk of testicular cancer.	III/B
◆ There is currently no evidence that early orchidopexy limits testicular cancer risk. Prospective evaluation of large numbers of men who have undergone orchidopexy by age two is required.	
◆ Acquired UDT probably explains the rise in incidence between age 5-11.	III/B
◆ Approximately 80% of primary acquired undescended testes descend spontaneously at puberty with appropriate testicular volumes for age. Therefore, watchful waiting until puberty is reasonable.	III/B

References

1. Fonkalsrud EW. In: *The Undescended Testis*. Fonkalsrud EW, Mengel W. Year Book Medical Publishers, Inc. Chicago, London, 1981: 1-4.
2. Hunter J. *The complete works of John Hunter F.R.S.* (p.41) Palmer, Philadelphia, 1841.
3. Cooper ERA. The histology of the retained testis in the human subject at different ages, and its comparison with the scrotal testis. *J Anat* 1929; 64: 5-27.
4. Backhouse KM. Embryology of the normal and cryptorchid testis. In: *The Undescended Testis*. Fonkalsrud EW, Mengel W. Year Book Medical Publishers, Inc. Chicago, London, 1981: 5-29.
5. Scorer CG. The incidence of incomplete descent of the testicle at birth. *Arch Dis Child* 1956; 31: 198-202.
6. John Radcliffe Hospital Cryptorchidism Study Group. Cryptorchidism: a prospective study of 7500 consecutive male births, 1984-8. *Arch Dis Child* 1992; 67: 892-899.
7. Hack WW, Meijer RW, van der Voort-Doedens LM, Bos SD, Haasnoot K. Natural course of acquired undescended testis in boys. *Br J Surg* 2003; 90(6): 728-31.
8. Hack WW, Meijer RW, Bos SD, Haasnoot K. A new clinical classification for undescended testis. *Scand J Urol Nephrol* 2003; 37(1): 43-7.
9. Donnell SC, Rickwood AMK, Jee LD, Jackson M. Congenital testicular maldescent: significance of the complete hernial sac. *Br J Urol* 1995; 75: 702-703.
10. American Academy of Paediatrics. Timing of elective surgery on the genitalia of male children with particular reference to the risks, benefits and psychological effects of surgery and anesthesia. *Pediatrics* 1996; 97: 590-594.
11. Kogan SJ. Fertility in cryptorchidism. An overview in 1987. *Eur J Pediatr* 1987; 146(Suppl 2): S21-S24.
12. Swerdlow AJ, Higgins CD, Pike MC. Risk of testicular cancer in a cohort of boys with cryptorchidism. *BMJ* 1997; 314: 1507-11.
13. Forman D, Pike MC, Davey G, Dawson S, Baker K, Chilvers CED, Oliver RTD, Coupland CAC. Aetiology of testicular

cancer: association with congenital abnormalities, age at puberty, infertility and exercise. *BMJ* 1994; 308: 1393-1399.

14. Gracia J, Gonzalez N, Gomez ME, Plaza L, Sanchez J, Alba J. Clinical and anatomopathological study of 2000 cryptorchid testes. *Br J Urol* 1995; 75: 697-701.

15. Kogan SJ, Fertility in Cryptorchidism in Hadziselimovic F. *Cryptorchidism, management and implications*. Springer Verlag, Berlin, 1983: 71-82.

16. Chilvers C, Dudley NE, Gough MH, Jackson MB, Pike MC. Undescended testis: the effect of treatment on subsequent risk of subfertility and malignancy. *J Pediatr Surg* 1986; 21(8): 691-6.

17. Lee PA, O'Leary LA, Songer NJ, Bellinger MF, LaPorte RE. Paternity after cryptorchidism: lack of correlation with age at orchidopexy. *Br J Urol* 1995; 75: 704-707.

18. Wilson-Storey D, McGenity K, Dickson JAS. Orchidopexy: the younger the better? *J R Coll Surg Edinb* 1990; 35: 362-364.

19. Mengel W, Zimmermann FA, Hecker WCH. Timing of repair for undescended testes. In: *The Undescended Testis*. Fonkalsrud EW, Mengel W. Year Book Medical Publishers Inc., Chicago, London, 1981: 170-183.

20. Hedinger CHR. Histological data in cryptorchidism. Cryptorchidism, diagnosis and treatment. *Paediatr Adolesc Endocrinol* 1979; 6: 3.

21. Hadziselimovic F, Herzog B, Seguchi H. Surgical correction of cryptorchidism at 2 years: electron microscopic and morphometric investigations. *J Pediatr Surg* 1975; 10: 19-26.

22. Mininberg DT, Rodger JC, Bedford JM. Ultrastructural evidence of the onset of testicular pathological conditions in the cryptorchid human testis within the first year of life. *J Urol* 1982; 128: 782-784.

23. Ludwig G, Potempa J. Der optimale zeitpunkt det behandlung des kryptorchismus. *Dtsch Med Wochenschr* 1975; 100: 680-683.

24. Kogan SJ, Tennenbaum S, Gill B, Reda E, Levitt SB. Efficacy of orchidopexy by patient age 1 year for cryptorchidism. *J Urol* 1990; 144: 508-509.

25. Puri P, O'Donnell B. Semen analysis of patients who had orchidopexy at or after seven years of age. *Lancet* 1988; 2(8619): 1051-2.

26. Chilvers C, Ansell P. Comment on orchidopexy at or after seven years of age. *Lancet* 1989; 1: 49.

27. Cromie WJ. Cryptorchidism and malignant testicular disease. In: *Cryptorchidism, management and implications*. Hadiselimovic F. Springer-Verlag, Berlin, 1983: 83-92.

28. Martin CD. Malignancy and the undescended testis. In: *The Undescended Testis*. Fonkalsrud EW, Mengel W. Year Book Medical Publishers Inc., Chicago, London, 1981: 144-156.

29. Chilvers C, Pike MC. Cancer risk in the undescended testicle. *Eur Urol Update Series* 1992; 1: 74-79.

30. Pike MC, Chilvers C, Peckham MJ. Effect of age at orchidopexy on risk of testicular cancer. *Lancet* 1986; 1(8492): 1246-8.

31. Giwercman A, Grinsted J, Hansen B, Jensen OM, Skakkebaek NE. Testicular cancer risk in boys with maldescended testes: a cohort study. *J Urol* 138: 1214-16.

32. Surana R, Puri P. Iatrogenic ascent of the testis: an under-recognized complication of inguinal hernia operation in children. *Br J Urol* 1994; 73: 580-581.

33. Atwell JD. Ascent of the testis: fact or fiction. *Br J Urol* 1985; 57: 474-477.

34. Robertson JFR, Azmy AF, Cochran W. Assent to ascent of the testis. *Br J Urol* 1988; 61: 146-147.

35. Colodny AH. Comment on iatrogenic ascent of the testis: an under-recognized complication of inguinal hernia operation in children. *Br J Urol* 1994; 74: 531.

Chapter 7

Timing of orchidopexy for undescended testes

Chapter 8

Varicocoele repair: does it work and how should we do it?

Gang Zhu MD PhD

Consultant Urologist [1]

Gordon Muir FRCS (Urol) FEBU

Consultant Urological Surgeon [2]

1 Beijing Hospital, Beijing, China
2 King's College Hospital, London, UK

Introduction

Varicocoele is a common condition seen in approximately 10%-15% of normal men on screening. Traditionally, it is taught that the problem is of a deficient valve at the junction of the left renal vein and the gonadal vein (the right gonadal vein draining in most cases straight to the inferior vena cava). While clinically often unilateral, there is ample evidence from observational studies that clinical examination is less than perfect in diagnosing varicocoele, missing many subclinical cases, particularly on the right side [1] **(III/B)**. Whether this matters is another question.

There are several methods to enhance the diagnostic accuracy of varicocoele which include Doppler ultrasound, scintigraphy, venography and contact thermography. We have been unable to find any studies which have rigorously compared the accuracy of these techniques. The vast majority of studies use scrotal Doppler ultrasound to detect retrograde pampiniform flow as an endpoint for confirmation of diagnosis and successful treatment. However, there is no good evidence to measure the accuracy of any technique in relation to its ability to detect or exclude clinically significant varicocoele.

Methodology

A number of areas in the treatment of varicocoele are controversial. To address these in an evidence-based way, a Medline and Cochrane database search was carried out over a ten-year period (1994-2004). All randomised studies and meta-analyses that could be found were included, as well as observational studies which fulfilled the following criteria:

- First description of a technique.
- Case series of 50 or more patients treated by one technique.
- Comparative studies of two techniques where the manuscript indicates a lack of selection between the patient groups (eg. consecutive case series vs consecutive historical controls).
- Studies with observational data on the pathophysiology of varicocoele.

Studies which were not clear in terms of the above, where the loss to follow-up rate was greater than 30% or where there appeared to be duplication of patient data with other published studies, were not considered.

Pathophysiology of varicocoele

The commonly held belief is of a "leaky valve" in the upper spermatic vein, but the spermatic vein in men with varicocoele has been shown to have poor intrinsic function compared to similar veins from patients without varicocoele [2]. This could cause either the classical valve dysfunction, or more general venous laxity.

In many mammals the testes are extracorporeal and slightly cooler than the core temperature: this is postulated as important for normal spermatogenesis. In varicocoele, excess veins around the testis seem to cause local heating of the organ, possibly affecting the contralateral testis, and indeed both testes do obtain temperature drop from varicocoele repair [3] **(IIb/B)**.

A few studies have looked at putative markers of oxidative stress in relation to variococoele, with Mostafa showing improvement in free radical concentrations following varicocoele repair. On a more directly functional note, Pierik's group noted an increase in both inhibin B and free androgen index following varicocoele repair in 30 men [4] **(IIb/B)**.

Symptoms of varicocoele

The three cardinal problems associated with varicocoele are pain, testicular atrophy and subfertility.

Pain

The cause of the pain is not well established, and while classical teaching leads us to expect a dull aching pain made worse by standing or sitting, no comparison has directly assessed pain character in relation to the extent or response to treatment of varicocoeles **(IV/C)**.

Hypotrophy or atrophy

Testicular hypotrophy or atrophy is commonly seen in young boys and adolescents with varicocoele. The overall rate of this is difficult to ascertain: some authors have either not noted testis hypotrophy or else have used differing methods (eg. ultrasound, physical examination, orchiometers) to gauge testis volume. Another problem in interpretation is having a reference range for unilateral hypotrophy in boys without varicocoele, since screening studies have tended to concentrate on diagnosing the varicocoele, then measuring the testicle in the affected group. Nonetheless, while there are no randomised studies, the evidence from a number of single arm and comparative studies is very uniform.

In every study reviewed which addressed the problem [5,6,7], there was evidence of "catch-up growth" in the majority of boys treated, with no reports of post-treatment testicular atrophy **(IIb/B)**. It may be that only clinical varicocoeles are worth treating in this respect [8]. Reversal of volume loss was not seen in one study addressing 61 adult men [9]. One study [10] attempted to match a small number of men who had varicocoeles treated in childhood and adolescence with age with untreated controls and found that the men who had been treated had better testis volumes and sperm counts. It has also been suggested that testicular hypotrophy is more commonly seen with larger varicocoeles [11,12] **(IIb/B)**.

Infertility

This is the most controversial area of varicocoele treatment. Men with infertility seem more than twice as likely as those in the general population to present with a clinical varicocoele. As well as testicular atrophy, large varicocoeles show an association with poor sperm quality and it has been suggested that the size of the varicocoele, as measured by vein diameter on ultrasound, may be of significance [13,14] **(IIb/B)**.

There are differing reports of problems attributed to varicocoele-related infertility, from azoospermia to motility problems alone. However, most authors describe a triad of low normal forms, poor motility and moderate oligospermia.

Randomised studies of varicocoele treatment for male factor infertility

In this area, a number of randomised trials have been attempted although none had a sham treatment arm, so no double blind trials are available. In some of these studies, conservative options such as scrotal cooling seem to have been used, while in others "counselling" was the alternative intervention.

Persistent night-time scrotal cooling does improve seminal parameters in men with varicocoele, but this must be assessed in the context of patient preference between regular and prolonged local treatment versus a single intervention [15] **(III/B)**.

A major defect in terms of assessing pregnancy results is that partner age was not assessed as a variable in most, and that follow-up was only carried out for a limited time.

A meta-analysis of these studies has been carried out [16] **(Ia/A)**, purporting to show no benefit in either patients with subclinical or clinical varicocoele. In fact, the treated group had a slightly higher rate of pregnancy (22% vs 19%) within a relatively short time frame, and semen parameters were improved for treated patients in most of the studies. In addition to patients with subclinical varicocoele, a number of men with completely normal semen analysis were included in this meta-analysis.

The authors conclude no benefit from treatment while accepting that subgroup analysis from these trials with differing entry criteria is unreliable. They suggest a control arm of ICSI in future studies, and also, that repeat semen analysis will tend to show regression towards the normal mean.

For randomised studies, recruitment seems to be a major issue, despite the very common nature of the problem. In a multicentre German study [17], only 67 patients were randomised to a study of sclerotherapy versus observation. The study was powered to need 460 randomised patients and was closed after three years. In this study, there were no significant differences in pregnancy rates at one year **(Ib/A)**, but the huge confidence intervals made the results hard to interpret.

As alluded to in the discussion of the Evers meta-analysis, a number of randomised studies have shown significant benefits from treatment after varicocoele repair but no significant pregnancy differences at one year, the usual reporting point [18,19]. Only one study has addressed longer-term outcomes, with significant benefits in both semen parameters and pregnancy rates at one year, the difference becoming more significant over the next 12 months [20]. Apart from the accepted need to wait a significant number of months to see spermogram improvements, it is reasonable to assume that men who have had surgery for varicocoele probably have a reduced number of conception attempts in the first few months postoperatviely due to pain.

In another study which randomised patients having laparoscopic repair between artery preservation and sacrifice, significant semen analysis improvements were seen in both groups but no intergroup difference was noted [21] **(Ib/A)**.

Another RCT looking at bilateral versus unilateral repair (for men with subclinical right varicocoele) showed significant and equal improvements in both groups [22] **(Ib/A)**.

There is thus conflicting data from the existing RCTs. It seems clear that many men can expect to see improvements in their semen analysis with varicocoele repair if they present with a palpable varicocoele and an abnormal sperm count. Counter-intuitively this does not seem to translate into a significant pregnancy improvement at one year. Longer follow-up might give a different answer.

Descriptive and non-randomised comparative studies [1,4,23-38,41,42] **(III/B)**

When non-randomised studies, and those studies using patients' own pre-treatment parameters as controls, are analysed, the results are strikingly different.

The data analysed from these papers relates to over 3,000 treated men from 21 different studies. In view of the generally high rate of clinical success in actually abolishing varicocoeles and the low complication rates (vide infra), no stratification of studies on the basis of varicocoele repair technique has been carried out. Embolisation, laparoscopic, microscopic and non-magnified open techniques are all represented in these studies.

These are a mixture of prospective and retrospective case series; all cases were, as far as can be ascertained from the literature, consecutive. But as stated in the introduction, papers in which a clear strategy to detect difference was not shown, were not included.

In all of these papers there was a significant improvement in motility and in normal forms in a proportion of patients. The smallest percentage of men to benefit in any study was 37% and the greatest, 86%. Overall, 65% of all men studied would appear to have improvements in seminal analysis. No significant decreases in sperm parameters are reported after treatment, nor are there any reports in these series of testicular atrophy or serious treatment-related complications.

Pregnancy rates are more difficult to analyse, since female factors are not fully explored and since in some papers the patients went on to IVF programmes within months of treatment. However, in those papers which do report spontaneous pregnancy (with a mean follow-up of around 13 months) the rates vary from 20%-48%. A number of authors find that couples can be raised from the position of requiring ICSI to intra-uterine insemination even if spontaneous fertility is not established.

Two large studies have addressed the relationship between varicocoele repair and assisted conception. In Ghent, 816 couples with a male factor problem were followed-up and compared according to treatment choice. In the men with varicocoele, intervention resulted in a 41% pregnancy rate compared with only 9% with counselling and timed intercourse [39]. In a meta-analysis done at Johns Hopkins Hospital in 1997 (looking at non-randomised controlled studies) it was concluded that the cost per delivery arising from varicocoele repair was likely to be less than half of that for an ICSI pregnancy in the same patient group [40].

Confounding factors in interpretation

The analysis of subclinical versus clinical varicocoeles is not always evident. In those studies which do clearly make the distinction there is a relatively consistent finding of no or little treatment benefit in men with subclinical varicocoele [41,42]. At the other end of the scale, men with decreased testicular volume and elevated FSH have been suggested to be less likely to benefit from physical treatment [13, 14]. While most studies did not include large numbers of patients with azoospermia, there are conflicting reports as to whether these patients are likely to benefit significantly from varicocoele repair [30, 32].

While not quantifiable, the cynic who has read this far and looked up the references might note that there seems to be more chance of urologists who examine this question finding great benefits from varicocoele repair, while those authors working in IVF units seem more likely to deem it a waste of time!

Why a different message from different types of study?

On the face of it, having a study which addresses a physical and objective parameter with regard to pre-treatment data has little to gain from randomisation, unless there is concern over biased patient selection. As none of the randomised studies was blinded to analysis (no sham treatment was included) the potential for placebo response and bias in analysis still exists.

Another problem with all of the studies addressed is the short follow-up in the context of fertility, and the lack of clarity in addressing female factors in the partner. This is particularly relevant in recommending strategies to couples where the female partner is older. The conventional wisdom seems that at least four months and possibly longer must elapse before a decision on seminal improvements can be made, but this seems to be based on knowledge of sperm maturation rather than longitudinal clinical studies.

As to the ability of future studies to address the place of varicocoele repair in male factor infertility, the inability of a large well designed multicentre RCT to approach recruitment targets must be borne in mind. The suggestion that any future studies should include an IVF control arm might be appealing to IVF units. However, the fact that many couples may be happy to take the chance of a minor definitive procedure with a moderate chance of success before committing themselves to the ICSI journey might scotch any such trial before it starts.

Overall, it seems that varicocoele repair is likely to improve sperm counts, motility and normal forms in infertile men who have clinical varicocoeles and no evidence of testicular failure as shown by testicular atrophy or FSH levels **(Ia/A and III/B)**. While it might seem bizarre to suggest that improving semen analysis parameters will not automatically improve fertility rates, there is debatable evidence as to whether pregnancy rates are improved. This may be due to the wrong questions having been asked (analysing men with normal sperm counts, azoospermia and too short follow-up).

Thus men, particularly those with a relatively elderly partner, should be made fully aware of scrotal cooling and IVF treatments as an alternative to varicocoele repair.

Varicocoele repair for pain [5, 43-48] (III/B)

Few studies report uniquely on men operated on for varicocoele pain. It was not possible to find any randomised trial comparing varicocoele repair with other techniques. Generally, authors seem to accept that the typical pain from varicocoele is a dull and persistent discomfort. In the studies reviewed where the treatment of pain was quantified, between 60%-85% of men were reported as being either pain-free or much improved following the procedure. No studies suggested a negative impact of varicocoele repair on scrotal pain.

Which technique? [5, 13, 28, 34, 43, 45, 49-59] (III/B)

As with many physical techniques, there are no clear randomised studies giving evidence of the

superiority of one technique over another. Individual and institutional skill is clearly important.

When assessing the differences between surgery and sclerotherapy, the general picture is one of sclerotherapy giving a higher initial failure rate and recurrence rate while allowing patients to recover and return to normal activity more quickly.

There is little convincing data to support the speed of return to normal activity for one or other surgical technique.

Several studies have purported to show increased patient preference for sclerotherapy but the interpretation of these data is not straightforward. Retrograde embolisation reports overall success rates (including initial failures) of 72%-81%, whereas for the antegrade Tauber technique, the rate is closer to 90% in most series. For ligation procedures most published authors are reporting long-term success rates of between 93%-99%. The fact that microsurgical techniques are often reported in the upper end of this range may relate either to the fact that it has superior efficacy or may reflect the large caseload being seen by those reporting data.

While many studies make much of the risk of postoperative testicular atrophy, this is hardly ever reported in published studies, so the risk with any technique appears well under 1%. Deliberate sacrifice of the testicular artery seems to do little to affect testis blood flow [60].

Hydrocoele can occur in the postoperative period, and again there is difficulty in interpreting results. It seems clear that many hydrocoeles are operated on quite quickly when other evidence suggests that the majority will resolve spontaneously given time. The risk of hydrocoele appears lowest with microsurgical approaches, with ligation and where lymphatic dye is combined with laparoscopy. However, persistent hydrocoele requiring surgery seems to be less than a 3%-5% risk with any procedure.

As with many variants of surgical procedures, local skill and enthusiasm will probably determine the optimal approach.

Chapter 8

Recommendations	Evidence level

- Varicocoele is common and associated with pain, as well as defects in testis and sperm development. — II/B

- Treatment improves a number of basic parameters such as temperature and oxidative stress. — II/B

- In the presence of unilateral testicular hypotrophy in children, repair of clinical varicocoele has a high chance of reversing volume loss. — II/B

- While one limited meta-analysis shows no pregnancy benefit for treatment of varicocoele-associated infertility, multiple observational studies suggest benefits. — I/A & III/B

- There may be a need to wait for more than 9-12 months to see a benefit in infertile men. Thus, infertile men with elderly partners should at least consider IVF/ICSI as an alternative. — IV/C

- Ideally, future studies looking at varicocoele in infertility should concentrate on men with abnormal sperm counts and clinical varicocoele. The use of control arms including IVF, and follow-up over two to three years, may be needed to be sure of outcome. We believe such trials will never recruit sufficient patients.

- Varicocoele repair seems effective for the treatment of associated pain in the majority of men. — III/B

- There is little evidence to support testicular artery preservation, or bilateral repair in the absence of bilateral clinical disease. — I/A

- Embolisation techniques seem less traumatic for the patient but with a slightly lower chance of success. No varicocoele repair technique is clearly superior and local expertise and availability should guide the patient's choice. — II & III/B

References

1. Gat Y, Bachar GN, Zukerman Z, Belenky A, Gornish M. Varicocele: a bilateral disease. *Fertil Steril* 2004; 81(2): 424-9.

2. Lund L, Ernst E, Sorensen HT, Oxlund H. Biomechanical properties of the internal spermatic vein in the normal population and patients with left-sided varicocele testis. *Eur Urol* 1998; 33(2): 233-7.

3. Wright EJ, Young GP, Goldstein M. Reduction in testicular temperature after varicocelectomy in infertile men. *Urology* 1997; 50(2): 257-9.

4. Pierik FH, Abdesselam SA, Vreeburg JT, Dohle GR, De Jong FH, Weber RF. Increased serum inhibin B levels after varicocele treatment. *Clin Endocrinol* (Oxf) 2001; 54(6): 775-80.

5. Greenfield SP, Seville P, Wan J. Experience with varicoceles in children and young adults. *J Urol* 2002; 168(4 Pt 2): 1684-8

6. Dattola P, Alberti A, Dattola A, Giannetto G, Basile G, Basile M. Inguino-crural hernias: preoperative diagnosis and post-operative follow-up by high-resolution ultrasonography. A personal experience. *Ann Ital Chir* 2002; 73(1): 65-8.

7. Lemack GE, Uzzo RG, Schlegel PN, Goldstein M. Microsurgical repair of the adolescent varicocele. *J Urol* 1998; 160(1): 179-81.

8. Culha M, Mutlu N, Acar O, Baykal M. Comparison of testicular volumes before and after varicocelectomy. *Urol Int* 1998; 60(4): 220-3.

9. Papanikolaou F, Chow V, Jarvi K, Fong B, Ho M, Zini A. Effect of adult microsurgical varicocelectomy on testicular volume. *Urology* 2000; 56(1): 136-9.

10. Sayfan J, Siplovich L, Koltun L, Benyamin N. Varicocele treatment in pubertal boys prevents testicular growth arrest. *J Urol* 1997; 157(4): 1456-7.

11. Sigman M, Jarow JP. Ipsilateral testicular hypotrophy is associated with decreased sperm counts in infertile men with varicoceles. *J Urol* 1997; 158(2): 605-7.

12. Thomas JC, Elder JS. Testicular growth arrest and adolescent varicocele: does varicocele size make a difference? *J Urol* 2002; 168(4 Pt 2): 1689-91.

13. Fujisawa M, Dobashi M, Yamasaki T, Okada H, Arakawa S, Kamidono S. Therapeutic strategy after microsurgical varicocelectomy in the modern assisted reproductive technology era. *Urol Res* 2002; 30(3): 195-8. Epub 2002 Jun 04.

14. Yoshida K, Kitahara S, Chiba K, Horiuchi S, Horimi H, Sumi S, Moriguchi H. Predictive indicators of successful varicocele repair in men with infertility. *Int J Fertil Womens Med* 2000; 45(4): 279-84.

15. Jung A, Eberl M, Schill WB. Improvement of semen quality by nocturnal scrotal cooling and moderate behavioural change to reduce genital heat stress in men with oligoasthenoterato-zoospermia. *Reproduction* 2001; 121(4): 595-603.

16. Evers JL, Collins JA. Assessment of efficacy of varicocele repair for male subfertility: a systematic review. *Lancet* 2003; 361(9372): 1849-52.

17. Krause W, Muller HH, Schafer H, Weidner W. Does treatment of varicocele improve male fertility? results of the "Deutsche Varikozelenstudie", a multicentre study of 14 collaborating centres. *Andrologia* 2002; 34(3): 164-71.

18. Yamamoto M, Hibi H, Hirata Y, Miyake K, Ishigaki T. Effect of varicocelectomy on sperm parameters and pregnancy rate in patients with subclinical varicocele: a randomized prospective controlled study. *J Urol* 1996; 155(5): 1636-8.

19. Nieschlag E, Hertle L, Fischedick A, Behre HM. Treatment of varicocele: counselling as effective as occlusion of the vena spermatica. *Hum Reprod* 1995; 10(2): 347-53.

20. Madgar I, Weissenberg R, Lunenfeld B, Karasik A, Goldwasser B. Controlled trial of high spermatic vein ligation for varicocele in infertile men. *Fertil Steril* 1995; 63(1): 120-4.

21. Yamamoto M, Tsuji Y, Ohmura M, Hibi H, Miyake K. Comparison of artery-ligating and artery-preserving varicocelectomy: effect on post-operative spermatogenesis. *Andrologia* 1995; 27(1): 37-40.

22. Grasso M, Lania C, Castelli M, Galli L, Rigatti P. Bilateral varicocele: impact of right spermatic vein ligation on fertility. *J Urol* 1995; 153(6): 1847-8.

23. Hsieh ML, Chang PL, Huang ST, Wang TM, Tsui KH. Loupe-assisted high inguinal varicocelectomy for sub-fertile men with varicoceles. *Chang Gung Med J* 2003; 26(7): 479-84.

24. Kibar Y, Seckin B, Erduran D. The effects of subinguinal varicocelectomy on Kruger morphology and semen parameters. *J Urol* 2002; 168(3): 1071-4.

25. Fujisawa M, Dobashi M, Yamasaki T, Okada H, Arakawa S, Kamidono S. Therapeutic strategy after microsurgical varicocelectomy in the modern assisted reproductive technology era. *Urol Res* 2002; 30(3): 195-8.

26. Maghraby HA. Laparoscopic varicocelectomy for painful varicoceles: merits and outcomes. *J Endourol* 2002; 16(2): 107-10.

27. Cayan S, Erdemir F, Ozbey I, Turek PJ, Kadioglu A, Tellaloglu S. Can varicocelectomy significantly change the way couples use assisted reproductive technologies? *J Urol* 2002; 167(4): 1749-52.

28. Jungwirth A, Gogus C, Hauser G, Gomahr A, Schmeller N, Aulitzky W, Frick J. Clinical outcome of microsurgical subinguinal varicocelectomy in infertile men. *Andrologia* 2001; 33(2): 71-4.

29. Kamal KM, Jarvi K, Zini A. Microsurgical varicocelectomy in the era of assisted reproductive technology: influence of initial semen quality on pregnancy rates. *Fertil Steril* 2001; 75(5): 1013-6.

30. Matkov TG, Zenni M, Sandlow J, Levine LA. Preoperative semen analysis as a predictor of seminal improvement following varicocelectomy. *Fertil Steril* 2001; 75(1): 63-8.

31. Scherr D, Goldstein M. Comparison of bilateral versus unilateral varicocelectomy in men with palpable bilateral varicoceles. *J Urol* 1999; 162(1): 85-8.

32. Matthews GJ, Matthews ED, Goldstein M. Induction of spermatogenesis and achievement of pregnancy after microsurgical varicocelectomy in men with azoospermia and severe oligoasthenospermia. *Fertil Steril* 1998; 70(1): 71-5.

33. Segenreich E, Israilov SR, Shmueli J, Niv E, Servadio C. Correlation between semen parameters and retrograde flow into the pampiniform plexus before and after varicocelectomy. *Eur Urol* 1997; 32(3): 310-4.

34. Feneley MR, Pal MK, Nockler IB, Hendry WF. Retrograde embolization and causes of failure in the primary treatment of varicocele. *Br J Urol* 1997; 80(4): 642-6.

35. Seftel AD, Rutchik SD, Chen H, Stovsky M, Goldfarb J, Desai N. Effects of subinguinal varicocele ligation on sperm concentration, motility and Kruger morphology. *J Urol* 1997; 158(5): 1800-3.

36. Parikh FR, Kamat SA, Kodwaney GG, Balaiah D. Computer-assisted semen analysis parameters in men with varicocele: is surgery helpful? *Fertil Steril* 1996; 66(3): 440-5.

37. Ferguson JM, Gillespie IN, Chalmers N, Elton RA, Hargreave TB. Percutaneous varicocele embolization in the treatment of infertility. *Br J Radiol* 1995l; 68(811): 700-3.

38. Tan SM, Ng FC, Ravintharan T, Lim PH, Chng HC. Laparoscopic varicocelectomy: technique and results. *Br J Urol* 1995; 75(4): 523-8.

39. Comhaire F, Milingos S, Liapi A, Gordts S, Campo R, Depypere H, Dhont M, Schoonjans F. The effective cumulative pregnancy rate of different modes of treatment of male infertility. *Andrologia* 1995; 27(4): 217-21

40. Schlegel PN. Is assisted reproduction the optimal treatment for varicocele-associated male infertility? A cost-effectiveness analysis. *Urology* 1997; 49(1): 83-90.

41. Jarow JP, Ogle SR, Eskew LA. Seminal improvement following repair of ultrasound detected subclinical varicoceles. *J Urol* 1996; 155(4): 1287-90.

42. Takahara M, Ichikawa T, Shiseki Y, Nakamura T, Shimazaki J. Relationship between grade of varicocele and the response to varicocelectomy. *J Urol* 1996; 3(4): 282-5.

43. Yeniyol CO, Tuna A, Yener H, Zeyrek N, Tilki A. High ligation to treat pain in varicocele. *Int Urol Nephrol* 2003; 35(1): 65-8.

44. Maghraby HA. Laparoscopic varicocelectomy for painful varicoceles: merits and outcomes. *J Endourol* 2002; 16(2): 107-10.

45. Ribe N, Manasia P, Sarquella J, Grimaldi S, Pomerol JM. Clinical follow-up after subinguinal varicocele ligation to treat pain. *Ital Urol Androl* 2002; 74(2): 51-3.

46. Cayan S, Kadioglu A, Orhan I, Kandirali E, Tefekli A, Tellaloglu S. The effect of microsurgical varicocelectomy on serum follicle stimulating hormone, testosterone and free

Chapter 8

testosterone levels in infertile men with varicocele. *BJU Int* 1999; 84(9): 1046-9.

47. Peterson AC, Lance RS, Ruiz HE. Outcomes of varicocele ligation done for pain. *J Urol* 1998; 159(5): 1565-7.

48. Lukkarinen O, Hellstrom P, Leinonen S, Juntunen K. Is varicocele treatment useful? *Ann Chir Gynaecol* 1997; 86(1): 40-4.

49. Itoh K, Suzuki Y, Yazawa H, Ichiyanagi O, Miura M, Sasagawa I. Results and complications of laparoscopic Palomo varicocelectomy. *Arch Androl* 2003; 49(2): 107-10.

50. Thomas JC, Elder JS. Testicular growth arrest and adolescent varicocele: does varicocele size make a difference? *J Urol* 2002; 168(4 Pt 2): 1689-91.

51. Cayan S, Akbay E, Bozlu M, Doruk E, Erdem E, Acar D, Ulusoy E. The effect of varicocele repair on testicular volume in children and adolescents with varicocele. *J Urol* 2002; 168(2): 731-4.

52. Alqahtani A, Yazbeck S, Dubois J, Garel L. Percutaneous embolization of varicocele in children: a Canadian experience. *J Pediatr Surg* 2002; 37(5): 783-5.

53. Ficarra V, Porcaro AB, Righetti R, Cerruto MA, Pilloni S, Cavalleri S, Malossini G, Artibani W. Antegrade scrotal sclerotherapy in the treatment of varicocele: a prospective study. *BJU Int* 2002; 89(3): 264-8.

54. Varlet F, Becmeur F; Groupe d'Etudes en Coeliochirurgie Infantile. Laparoscopic treatment of varicoceles in children. Multicentric prospective study of 90 cases. *Eur J Pediatr Surg* 2001; 11(6): 399-403.

55. Mazzoni G. Adolescent varicocele: treatment by antegrade sclerotherapy. *J Pediatr Surg* 2001; 36(10): 1546-50.

56. Esposito C, Monguzzi G, Gonzalez-Sabin MA, Rubino R, Montinaro L, Papparella A, Esposito G, Settimi A, Mastroianni L, Zamparelli M, Sacco R, Amici G, Damiano R, Innaro N. Results and complications of laparoscopic surgery for pediatric varicocele. *J Pediatr Surg* 2001; 36(5): 767-9.

57. Poddoubnyi IV, Dronov AF, Kovarskii SL, Korznikova IN, Darenkov IA, Zalikhin DV. Laparoscopic ligation of testicular veins for varicocele in children. A report of 180 cases. *Surg Endosc* 2000; 14(12): 1107-9.

58. Kiilholma P, Nikkanen V, Nurmi M, Satokari K. Percutaneous sclerotherapy for varicocele embolization. *Tech Urol* 1998; 4(1): 18-21.

59. Bigot JM, Le Blanche AF, Carette MF, Gagey N, Bazot M, Boudghene FP. Anastomoses between the spermatic and visceral veins: a retrospective study of 500 consecutive patients. *Abdom Imaging* 1997; 22(2): 226-32.

60. Student V, Zatura F, Scheinar J, Vrtal R, Vrana J. Testicle hemodynamics in patients after laparoscopic varicocelectomy evaluated using color Doppler sonography. *Eur Urol* 1998; 33(1): 91-3.

Chapter 9

Investigation of men with erectile dysfunction

Ian Eardley MA MChir FRCS (Urol) FEBU
Consultant Urologist
Omer Baldo MB BS MRCS (Glas)
Clinical Research Fellow, Urology

ST JAMES' UNIVERSITY HOSPITAL, LEEDS, UK

Introduction

Appropriate evaluation of patients with erectile dysfunction (ED) is important for a number of reasons. The first is to confirm the diagnosis of ED (as opposed to disorders of drive or ejaculation) and this is usually best done by means of a detailed sexual history. The second is to ascertain the severity of the problem and this can be performed objectively with questionnaires (eg. International Index of Erectile Function - IIEF) or it can be ascertained from the history. The third is to identify treatable conditions that may be relevant to the aetiology of the ED such as diabetes, hyperlipidaemia, depression, hypertension, or hypogonadism. Some of these conditions will be identified during history and examination while some will be identified by special investigations. The fourth objective is to identify patients who have causes of ED that might be amenable to specific treatment, such as men with vascular anomalies amenable to reconstructive surgery, men with endocrine abnormalities amenable to specific therapy and men with a psychogenic component amenable to therapy.

The conventional approach then to most men presenting with ED is a combination of history, physical examination and special investigations. In the context of determining the level of evidence that is available in the literature to support these interventions, we have considered the levels of evidence available to support each of the three parts of the assessment in the attainment of the four objectives outlined above.

What role does the clinical history play in the assessment of erectile dysfunction?

The clinical history is traditionally held to be the cornerstone in establishing the diagnosis of ED. The aims are to establish the nature of the problem, its chronology and severity, to identify psychosexual elements and possible organic causes, to explore any relationship issues and to ascertain the expectations of the patient and (where possible) his partner. Most of the evidence to support the role of the history comes from Expert Committee Reports, such as those published following the 1st and 2nd International Consultation on Erectile Dysfunction [1, 2] **(IV/C)**.

There are a number of issues relating to the clinical history that have been investigated in the literature as outlined below.

Is it possible to differentiate organic from psychogenic ED?

From a physician's perspective, an attempt to differentiate between the psychogenic and the organic causes of ED is of some value. While the common consensus holds that in most men, there are usually a mixture of organic and psychogenic factors that have resulted in ED, the identification of men with predominantly psychogenic ED might be expected to direct therapy, with consideration being given to psychosexual counselling. There is evidence to suggest that psychogenic ED is likely to have an acute onset, that it is likely to be situational, that it is likely to have varying severity and that it is likely to be associated with rigid non-coital erections. In a study of 176 men with ED, a screening test based on the Leiden Impotence Questionnaire (LIQ) was tested to differentiate organic from psychogenic ED [3] **(III/B)**. A logistic regression model including six general items from the LIQ correctly identified psychogenic ED in 62% of cases and organic ED in 86%. These items were: sudden loss of erections (which if present was suggestive of psychogenic); presence of morning erections (which if present was suggestive of psychogenic); rigidity of morning erections (which if present was suggestive of psychogenic); decline in sexual interest (which if present was suggestive of organic); ED due to psychological problems (in the opinion of the patient) (which if present was suggestive of psychogenic); reduced size of penis (which if present was suggestive of organic).

A prior study had also demonstrated the value of assessing non-coital erections [4] **(III/B)**. In a study of 32 patients, Segraves *et al*, demonstrated the value of early morning erections, masturbatory erections and non-coital erections as a means of identifying cases of psychogenic ED.

Is it possible to assess the severity of ED?

A commonly held view is that mild ED is characterised by difficulties in maintaining an erection, and that as the condition becomes more severe, then there is difficulty in initiating an erection, which then progresses until the man gets no erections at all. There is no direct evidence to support this common observation although recent epidemiological studies have shown that these issues correlate well with the patient's perception of whether the ED is severe or not. A large epidemiological study of 2912 men with ED explored this issue of severity [5] **(III/B)**. Men who believed their ED to be severe (as opposed to moderate or mild) were more likely to get no erection at all and were also more likely to view their problem as permanent, while men with mild ED were more likely to have trouble maintaining their erections, and were more likely to view their problem as being temporary.

The introduction of validated questionnaires to assess sexual function has also aided the assessment of disease severity and these are discussed below.

What is the role of validated questionnaires in the assessment of men with ED?

In recent years a number of questionnaires have been developed to assess sexual function. While the initial impetus to develop some of these questionnaires came from new developments in therapy for ED, the questionnaires do now provide an objective means of both assessing disease severity and assessing response to therapy.

The most important of these questionnaires is the International Index of Erectile Function (IIEF). Rosen *et al* [6] developed this self-administered 15-item questionnaire in 1997, and it can be divided into five domains, namely erectile function, orgasmic function, sexual drive, intercourse satisfaction and overall satisfaction. The instrument has been well validated and has been adopted widely as an investigative tool. It is psychometrically sound and easy to administer in research and clinical settings. The Erectile Function domain of the IIEF has been extensively used in clinical trials of PDE5 inhibitors [7, 8, 9] and has become one of the most valuable means of assessing response to therapy.

A five-item version of the IIEF has been developed and evaluated as a screening test for ED [10]. The authors identified and validated five levels of severity:

severe (score 5-7); moderate (score 8-11); mild to moderate (score 12-16); mild (score 17-21); no ED (score 22-25). The EF domain of the IIEF (which includes six questions of the IIEF) has been used in a similar way, and recent publications have correlated the EF domain score with the percentage of successful intercourse attempts [11].

An alternative validated questionnaire is the Brief Male Sexual Function Inventory (BMSFI) that assesses sexual drive, erections, ejaculation, problem assessment and overall satisfaction [12]. It has been utilised much less extensively, and its ability to assess disease severity or the response to therapy is less clear.

Other questionnaires that have been recently developed and validated include the Self Esteem and Relationship (SEAR) questionnaire as an instrument to assess psychosocial variables in men with ED [13], the Psychological and Interpersonal Relationship Scales (PAIRS) that is a disease-specific quality of life questionnaire [14], and the Erectile Dysfunction Index of Treatment Satisfaction (EDITS) which assesses satisfaction with treatment [15]. Although all have been used in the context of clinical trials of therapies for ED, their value in assessing either disease severity or response to therapy is currently unclear.

What role does the physical examination play in the assessment of men with ED?

The physical examination has no role in the diagnosis of ED or in the assessment of ED severity. It should have a role in the identification of comorbid risk factors that might have contributed to the ED. It is generally accepted that for most patients a full general examination is unnecessary and that a focused examination is appropriate although there is disagreement about the extent of this examination. The Expert Committee Reports, published following the 1st and 2nd International Consultation on Erectile Dysfunction [1,2], suggested that the following were appropriate: complete genital examination (including digital rectal examination); assessment of gynaecomastia; assessment of body hair and fat distribution; assessment of blood pressure, heart rate, peripheral pulses and peripheral oedema; assessment

of vibratory sensation and bulbocavernosus reflex; and assessment of lower limb strength and coordination. Other groups have recommended a more focused examination with only blood pressure measurement, assessment of secondary sexual characteristics and examination of the genitalia (excluding digital rectal examination) being mandatory in all cases [16, 17].

What role does laboratory investigation play in the assessment of men with ED?

Laboratory investigation has no role in the diagnosis of ED, nor in the assessment of severity of ED. Currently its primary role is in the identification of risk factors for ED, that might require specific treatment in their own right, or that might be amenable to specific treatment which in turn might lead to the cure of the ED. The main issues to be considered to be relevant here are the diagnosis of diabetes, the diagnosis of dyslipidaemia and the diagnosis of endocrine disorders.

Diagnosis of diabetes

Diabetes is one of the commoner causes of erectile dysfunction. The pathophysiology of ED in diabetics is complex, and involves vascular and neurological changes together with endothelial and smooth muscle dysfunction. Consensus statements confirm the value of diagnosing diabetes in men who present with ED [1, 2, 16, 17, 18], and there are a number of publications which confirm that ED can be the presenting symptom of diabetes [19, 20]. In the former study of 497 men who had been referred for assessment of their erectile dysfunction, 11.1% were found to suffer from undiagnosed diabetes mellitus while a further 4.2% had impaired glucose tolerance [19]. In the latter study, the prevalence of known diabetes was 17% in a group of men presenting with ED, and the prevalence of undiagnosed diabetes was 4.7%. A further 3.7% had an abnormal fasting blood sugar, suggesting impaired glucose tolerance [20].

The crucial issue is how best to screen for diabetes? The options include urinalysis, random blood sugar, fasting blood sugar, the HbA1c and the oral glucose tolerance test (OGTT). The latter is the gold standard, but impracticable as a screening test. The WHO have suggested that the fasting blood sugar is the most appropriate screening test, with a cut-off at 7mmol/l [21], and there is evidence to support this. Mannucci et al [22], in a study of 1215 adults without previously known diabetes, assessed the sensitivity and specificity of Fasting Blood Sugar and HbA1c in diagnosing diabetes, with OGTT as standard. They found that fasting blood sugar, with a threshold of 7.0mmol/l, appeared to be sufficient for the screening and diagnosis of diabetes. Within the context of screening men with ED, fasting blood glucose was demonstrated to be superior to urinalysis in the diagnosis of ED, with the latter having a sensitivity of only 20% [20].

Diagnosis of dyslipidaemia

While dyslipidaemia is generally recognised as a risk factor for cardiovascular disease and has been shown to be epidemiologically associated with ED [23], the value of testing for dyslipidaemia in men presenting with ED has not been extensively investigated. Expert panels have recommended that lipids be measured in men presenting with ED for some years [1], but the evidence to support this contention has been lacking until recently.

In a study of 215 consecutive men presenting with ED and 100 potent controls, a fasting lipid screen which included total cholesterol (TC), triglycerides, HDL-cholesterol and LDL-cholesterol, was used to identify dyslipidaemia [24]. Significant differences in TC, HDL cholesterol and the ratio of TC/HDL cholesterol were identified. Multivariate analysis demonstrated patient age, TC and TC/HDL cholesterol to be important independent predictors of ED. Perhaps the most important finding was the suggestion that the men who presented with ED had a significantly greater calculated risk of coronary heart disease than the controls.

Diagnosis of endocrine disease

Although endocrine disorders are an uncommon cause of erectile dysfunction, they are potentially significant in that treatment of the underlying endocrine abnormality can sometimes cure the ED. The endocrine disorders that can lead to ED are

hypogonadism, hyperprolactinaemia and thyroid disease. Consensus statements support routine testing for hypogonadism but usually view testing for prolactin and thyroid dysfunction as optional [1]. However, the evidence to support these recommendations is mixed and controversial.

It is generally agreed that if clinical evaluation reveals decreased libido, testicular atrophy, abnormal secondary sexual characteristics of gynaecomastia then a complete endocrine evaluation is warranted. However, the appropriate endocrine screen for the man with simple erectile dysfunction remains controversial. One study of 508 consecutive men presenting with ED identified a 15.6% prevalence of hypogonadism and a 1.8% prevalence of hyperprolactinaemia [25]. The authors concluded that routine endocrine screening remains a necessary part of the evaluation for sexual dysfunction. A further study of 1022 patients with ED [26] identified a prevalence of hypogonadism of 4% in men aged under 50 years and 9% in men aged over 50 years. They identified only one prolactin-secreting tumour. The authors concluded that routine endocrine testing could not be justified in all men. However, they also found that screening only those men with low desire would have missed 40% of the cases of low testosterone, and concluded (perhaps arbitrarily) that under the age of 50 years, testosterone screening was only justified in those with ED and low desire, while over the age of 50 years, it was justified in all men. Prolactin levels were only to be assessed in men with low sexual desire, gynaecomastia and/or a low testosterone.

There are a number of practical issues. Testosterone should be measured in the morning, since there is a diurnal fall of perhaps 30% in the afternoon. If the testosterone is abnormal on initial testing, it should be repeated, together with assays for prolactin, Luteinising Hormone (LH) and Follicular Stimulating Hormone (FSH). In one of the studies described above, the second testosterone assay was normal in 60%.

Finally, there is a great deal of debate about the optimal testosterone assay with the options being total testosterone, free testosterone or bioavailable testosterone. Testosterone exists in three different forms in plasma: free, albumin-bound and bound to sex hormone binding globulin (SHBG). Ninety-eight percent of testosterone is bound to plasma protein, with most of the binding (57%) to SHBG and 40% to albumin. Total testosterone can be affected by changes in the SHBG, but is the easiest (and cheapest) assay to perform. It is certainly the test that is used most widely. The free testosterone is the most important biologically, but the assay is very much more expensive and more open to technical inaccuracy. The bioavailable testosterone is the combined free and albumin-bound testosterone and can be calculated with knowledge of the total testosterone and SHBG levels. Accordingly, the recommendation is that if cost is not an issue, then free testosterone should be measured [1]. If cost is an issue, then total testosterone should be measured together with SHBG.

What is the role of specialised vascular testing in the assessment of men with ED?

In the late 1980s and early 1990s, vascular assessment was performed in all patients with ED at presentation. With the advent of effective oral therapies for ED, most consensus statements now reserve vascular investigations for those men in whom there might be a vascular cause that would be amenable to specific therapy [1]. Essentially, this means that vascular testing is reserved for the selection of patients for vascular surgery. Currently, the main group of patients in whom vascular surgery can be justified are young men with ED secondary to traumatic damage to penile arteries. Although the commonest cause of injury is pelvic or perineal trauma, there is recent evidence to suggest that men who have developed ED secondary to bicycle riding might also benefit from vascular reconstructive surgery. Occasionally, vascular testing is helpful in reassuring patients that there is no significant vascular cause, and it may also be of occasional value in medicolegal cases.

Initial testing is usually performed with duplex ultrasound scanning of the penile arteries under conditions of maximal smooth muscle relaxation. This is usually achieved by intracavernosal injection of alprostadil or by visual sexual stimulation, or both. The usual parameters measured are the peak systolic blood flow velocity (PSV), and the end diastolic velocity (EDV). For men with normal erectile function, the mean PSV has been measured at 34.8cm/sec [27],

40cm/sec [28] and 47cm/sec [29]. All three studies suggested that a PSV less than 25cm/sec was indicative of vascular disease, while a further study demonstrated that this cut-off value had a sensitivity of 100% and a specificity of 95% [30] in the diagnosis of vasculogenic ED.

Internal pudendal arteriography is usually reserved for young men with abnormal duplex findings who are candidates for reconstructive vascular surgery [1].

Assessment of the veno-occlusive mechanism is intended to assess smooth muscle function, which is crucial for veno-occlusion to occur. Duplex scanning can be used as a screen for this, with an EDV greater than 3cms/sec having a sensitivity of 69% and a specificity of 94% [30]. The gold standard assessment for veno-occlusive dysfunction remains penile cavernosography and cavernosometry, although it is performed much less frequently than was the case when venous ligation was being used as a treatment for ED. Nowadays, its use is reserved for those cases where there is a site-specific venous leak in patients in whom vascular surgery is considered to be a treatment option [1]. Such cases include congenital venous leak, venous leak secondary to Peyronie's disease and cases secondary to penile fracture. As with duplex scanning, maximal smooth muscle relaxation is required, and the most important measure is thought to be the flow required to maintain an erection. Normally, this should be 3ml/sec or less and maintenance flow rates higher than this are thought to indicate abnormal venous leakage (or incomplete smooth muscle relaxation) [1].

What is the place of other tests in men with ED?

Nocturnal penile tumescence (NPT) is a normal phenomenon whereby men develop an erection four to six times per night. While assessment of nocturnal erections was used previously to identify men with psychogenic ED (where nocturnal erections are preserved), it is now rarely used other than as a research tool. Similarly, assessment of the erectile response to visual stimulation with a machine designed to record changes in penile girth and tumescence (the Rigiscan® machine) is also used principally as a research tool.

Chapter 9

Recommendations	Evidence level

What role does the clinical history play in the assessment of men with erectile dysfunction?

◆ History is valuable in the diagnosis of ED.	IV/C
◆ History is valuable is assessing severity of ED.	III/B
◆ Symptom scores are valuable in assessing severity of ED.	Ib/A
◆ Symptom scores are valuable in assessing response to therapy.	Ib/A
◆ History is valuable in differentiating psychogenic from organic ED.	III/B
◆ History is valuable in identifying relevant risk factors for ED.	IV/C
◆ History is valuable in identifying patients suitable for specialist investigation and treatment.	IV/C

What role does the physical examination play in the assessment of men with ED?

◆ There is general acceptance that the physical examination has no role in the diagnosis of ED, in differentiating organic from psychogenic ED, or in assessing severity of ED.	
◆ Physical examination is valuable in identifying relevant risk factors for ED.	IV/C

What role does laboratory investigation play in the assessment of men with ED?

◆ There is consensus that the diagnosis of diabetes is important in men with ED.	IIb/B
◆ Diabetes is more commonly found in men with ED.	IIb/B
◆ Fasting blood sugar is the optimal method of diagnosing diabetes.	IIb/B
◆ There is consensus that diagnosis of dyslipidaemia is important in men with ED.	IIb/B
◆ Dyslipidaemia is more commonly found in men with ED.	IIb/B
◆ A fasting lipid screen is the optimal method of diagnosing dyslipidaemia.	IIb/B
◆ There is consensus that the diagnosis of hypogonadism is important in men with ED.	IV/C
◆ There is no consensus as to the most appropriate assay. Most clinicians use either total testosterone, free testosterone of bioavailable testosterone.	
◆ There is no consensus as to the value of screening for hyperprolactinaemia.	
◆ There is consensus that routine investigation of thyroid disease is unnecessary in men with ED.	IV/C

What is the role of vascular assessment in men with ED?

◆ There is consensus that vascular testing is inappropriate in most men with ED.	IV/C
◆ There is the assessment that duplex ultrasound scanning is the most valuable vascular investigation in those men where vascular assessment is appropriate.	IV/C
◆ There is consensus that vascular assessment should be performed with maximal penile smooth muscle relaxation.	III/B

References

1. Jardin A, Wagner G, Khoury S, Giuliano F, Padma-Nathan H, Rosen R. *Erectile Dysfunction*. The 1st International Consultation on Erectile Dysfunction. Plymbridge, 2000.

2. Lue T, Giuliano F, Khoury, S, Rosen R. The 2nd International Consultation on Sexual Dysfunctions. Plymbridge, 2004.

3. Speckens AEM, Hengeveld MW, Lycklama A Nijeholt, Van Hemert AM, Hawton KE. Discrimination between psychogenic and organic erectile dysfunction. *J Psychosom Res* 1993; 37: 135-145.

4. Segraves KA, Segraves RT, Schoenberg HW. Use of the sexual history to differentiate organic from psychogenic impotence. *Arch Sex Behav* 1987; 16: 125-137.

5. Fisher WA, Rosen RC, Eardley I, Niederberger C, Nadel A, Kaufman J, Sand M. The Multinational Men's Attitudes to Life Events and Sexuality (MALES) Study: II: Understanding Treatment Seeking Patterns Among Men with Erectile Dysfunction. *J Sex Med* (in press).

6. Rosen RC, Riley A, Wagner G, Osterloh I, Kirkpatrick J, Mishra A. The international index of erectile function (IIEF): a multidimensional scale for assessment of erectile dysfunction. *Urology* 1997; 49: 822-830.

7. Goldstein I, Lue TF, Padma-Nathan H, Rosen RC, Steers WD, Wicker PA. Oral sildenafil in the treatment of erectile dysfunction. *N Engl J Med* 1998; 338: 1397-1404.

8. Brock GB, McMahon CG, Chen KK, *et al*. Efficacy and safety of tadalafil for the treatment of erectile dysfunction: results of integrated analyses. *J Urol* 2002; 168: 1332-6.

9. Hellstrom WJ, Gittelman M, Karlin G, Segerson T, Thibonnier M, Taylor T, Padma-Nathan H. Vardenafil for treatment of men with erectile dysfunction: efficacy and safety in a randomized, double-blind, placebo-controlled trial. *J Andrology* 2002; 23(6): 763-71.

10. Rosen RC, Cappelleri JC, Smith MD, Lipsky J, Pena BM. Development of evaluation of an abridged, 5-item version of the International Index of Erectile Function (IIEF-5) as a diagnostic tool for erectile dysfunction. *Int J Impo Res* 1999; 11: 319-326.

11. Padma-Nathan H, Montorsi F, Giuliano F, Meuleman EJH, Auerbach S, Eardley I, McCollough A, Homering M, and Segerson T for the North American and European Vardenafil Study Group. Vardenafil Restores Erectile Function to Normal Range in Men With Erectile Dysfunction. *Urology* (in press).

12. O'Leary M, Fowler F, Lenderking W, Barber B, Sagnier P, Guess H, Barry M. A brief male sexual function inventory for urology. *Urology* 1995; 46: 697-706.

13. Cappelleri JC, Althof SE, Siegel RL, Shpilsky A, Bell SS, Duttagupta S. Development and validation of the Self-Esteem and Relationship (SEAR) questionnaire in erectile dysfunction. *Int J Impo Res* 2004; 16: 30-38.

14. Swindle RW, Cameron AE, Lockhart DC, Rosen RC. The Psychological and Interpersonal Relationship Scales: assessing psychological and relationship outcomes with erectile dysfunction and its treatment. *Arch Sex Behav* 2004; 33: 19-30.

15. Althof SE, Corty EW, Levine SB, Burnett AL, *et al*. EDITS: development of questionnaires for evaluating satisfaction with treatments for erectile dysfunction. *Urology* 1999; 53: 793-799.

16. Ralph DJ, McNicholas T. UK management guidelines for Erectile Dysfunction. *BMJ* 2000; 321: 499-503.

17. Gingell C, Wright P, Barnes T, *et al*. Guidance on the management of erectile dysfunction in Primary Care. *Prescriber* 1999; 10 (Suppl): 1-16.

18. Montague DK, Barada JH, Belker AM, *et al*. Clinical guidelines on erectile dysfunction: summary report on the treatment of organic erectile dysfunction. The American Urological Asscoiation. *J Urol* 1996; 156: 2007-2011.

19. Maatman TJ, Montague DK, Martin LM. Erectile dysfunction in men with diabetes mellitus. *Urology* 1987; 29: 589-92.

20. Sairam K, Kulinskaya E. Boustead GB. Hanbury DC. McNicholas TA. Prevalence of undiagnosed diabetes mellitus in male erectile dysfunction. *BJU Int* 2001; 88: 68-71.

21. Alberti KG, Zimmet PZ. Definition, diagnosis and classification of diabetes mellitus and its complications. Part I: Diagnosis and Classification of Diabetes Mellitus. Provisional report of a WHO consultation. *Diabet Med* 1998; 15: 539-553.

22. Mannucci E, Ognibene A, Sposato I, Brogi M, Gallori G, Bardini G, Cremasco F, Messer G, Rotella C. Fasting plasma glucose and glycated haemoglobin in the screening of diabetes and impaired glucose tolerance. *Acta Diabeto* 2003; 40: 181-186.

23. Wei M, Macera C, Davis D, Hornung C, Nankin H, Blair S. Total cholesterol and high density lipoprotein cholesterol are important predictors of erectile dysfunction. *Am J Epidemiology* 1994; 140: 930-937.

24. Roumeguere TH, Wespes E, Carpentier Y, Hoffmann P, Schulman CC. Erectile dysfunction is associated with a high prevalence of hyperlipidaemia and coronary heart disease risk. *Eur Urology* 2003; 44: 355-359.

25. Govier F, McClure D, Kramer-Levien D. Endocrine screening of sexual dysfunction using free testosterone determination. *J Urol* 1996; 156: 405-408.

26. Buvat J, Lemaire A. Endocrine screening in 1,022 men with erectile dysfunction: clinical significance and cost-effectiveness strategy. *J Urol* 1997; 158: 1764-1767.

27. Broderick GA, Lue TF. The penile bloodflow study: evaluation of vasculogenic impotence. In: *Erectile Dysfunction*. Jonas U, Thon WF, Stief CG, Eds. Springer Verlag, 1991.

28. Shabsigh R, Fishman IJ, Shottland Y, *et al*. Comparison of penile duplex ultrasonography with nocturnal penile tumescence monitoring for the evaluation of erectile dysfunction. *J Urol* 1990; 924-927.

29. Benson CB, Vikers MA. Sexual impotence caused by vascular disease: diagnosis with duplex sonography. *Am J Roentgenol* 1989; 153: 1149.

30. Quam JP, King BF, James EM, Lewis RW, Brakke DM, Ilstrup DM, Parulkar BG, Hattery RR. Duplex and color Doppler sonographic evaluation of vasculogenic impotence. *Am J Roentgenol* 1989; 153: 1141-7.

Chapter 9

Chapter 9

Chapter 10

The treatment of chronic prostatitis/ chronic pelvic pain syndrome (CPPS)

G Richard D Batstone MA MB BChir MD FRCS (Urol)

Consultant Urologist

REDCLIFFE HOSPITAL, QUEENSLAND, AUSTRALIA

Introduction

Chronic prostatitis is a disorder with an uncertain aetiology. It is associated with a symptom complex consisting of pain in the perineum, testis, bladder, penis, pain on ejaculation and pain on urination. There is also disturbance of urination with primarily a feeling of incomplete emptying and frequent micturition. Prostatitis seems to be a common condition with a number of well conducted epidemiological studies citing incidence rates between 3-4/1000/year and prevalence rates between 9%-16% [1, 2, 3, 4] **(III/B)**. The sickness impact of chronic prostatitis is equivalent to that experienced by patients with myocardial infarction, angina and Crohn's disease [5] **(IIb/B)**. In a review article published in 2000, McNaughton Collins commented that there were no gold standard diagnostic tests or treatments for chronic abacterial prostatitis [6] **(Ia/A)**. Recent National Institutes of Health (NIH) sponsored initiatives are beginning to change this view and investigators have produced a number of grade A and B studies evaluating the diagnosis and treatment of men with chronic prostatitis/chronic pelvic pain syndrome. Still much about chronic prostatitis remains uncertain and the condition remains a diagnosis of exclusion, lacking both a gold standard diagnostic test and a gold standard treatment option.

This chapter will discuss the classification, aetiology, diagnosis, evaluation and treatment of prostatitis, with emphasis on the diagnosis and treatment of chronic prostatitis.

The classification of prostatitis

In 1995, researchers with an interest in the condition met under the auspices of the NIH. This meeting resulted in a new classification for prostatitis - the 1995 NIH classification [7]. The old terms "chronic abacterial prostatitis" and "prostatodynia" were discarded and re-termed chronic pelvic pain syndrome (CPPS) and subdivided into inflammatory and non-inflammatory CPPS. A new category was also made: type IV prostatitis or asymptomatic inflammatory prostatitis. Table 1 outlines the new classification system **(IV/C)**.

Chapter 10

Table 1. The 1995 NIH classification of prostatitis.

Type	Classification	Definition
I	Acute bacterial prostatitis	Evidence of acute bacterial infection
II	Chronic bacterial prostatitis	Evidence of recurrent bacterial infection
III	Chronic Pelvic Pain Syndrome (old abacterial prostatitis and prostatodynia)	Symptom duration for at least 3 months
IIIa	Inflammatory CPPS	White blood cells in semen, expressed prostatic secretions or after voided bladder 3 (sediment from initial 10ml urine after prostatic massage during Meares-Stamey 4 glass test)
IIIb	Non-inflammatory CPPS	No white blood cells in semen, expressed prostatic secretions or after voided bladder 3 (sediment from initial 10ml urine after prostatic massage during Meares-Stamey 4 glass test)
IV	Asymptomatic inflammatory prostatitis	No symptoms, incidental diagnosis during prostate biopsy or presence of white blood cells in prostatic secretions or semen during evaluation for other disorders

The differentiation between category II and category III prostatitis is based on the Stamey localisation [8] **(III/B)**. This paper describes longitudinal urinary bacterial localisation studies of four patients with chronic bacterial prostatitis (recurrent urinary tract infections). Figure 1 outlines this procedure. For the diagnosis of category II prostatitis the patient must have a culture of a standard uropathogen in the expressed prostatic secretions (EPS) or voided bladder specimen 3 (VB3) of at least 1 log greater in colony forming units/ml (CFU/ml) than that cultured in voided bladder specimen 1 (VB1) and the presence of inflammatory cells "localised" to the prostate (see below). Table 2 lists the standard uropathogens [9].

The differentiation of categories IIIa and IIIb CPPS is based on the finding of inflammatory cells in the EPS or VB3. The generally accepted limits are: >10 leucocytes/1000x field for the EPS, or >10 leucocytes /400x field on cyto-centrifuged VB3 [10], or >1x10^6 leukocytes/ml of semen [11] **(IV/C)**.

Problems with the classification

There are problems with this classification system. One should be wary of classifying a patient with symptoms of chronic prostatitis (pelvic pain and urinary symptoms) as having category II or chronic bacterial prostatitis for the following reasons. Nickel has demonstrated comparable responses to ofloxacin in his cohort of patients (with pelvic pain) diagnosed with category II and category III prostatitis on the basis of urine localisation studies [12]. Furthermore, if normal individuals undergo Stamey localisation the same percentage of them would be classified as type II prostatitis as a cohort of men with symptomatic chronic pelvic pain syndrome [13]. These studies are further evidence that bacteria are not pathogenic in this group of patients and cast doubt on the utility of the Stamey localisation in men with chronic pelvic pain **(IIa/B)**.

The differentiation between IIIa and IIIb CPPS is also problematic. "Normal" individuals have white blood cells (WBCs) in their EPS in comparable levels to those diagnosed with non-specific urethritis and chronic prostatitis [14]. Patients with CPPS do,

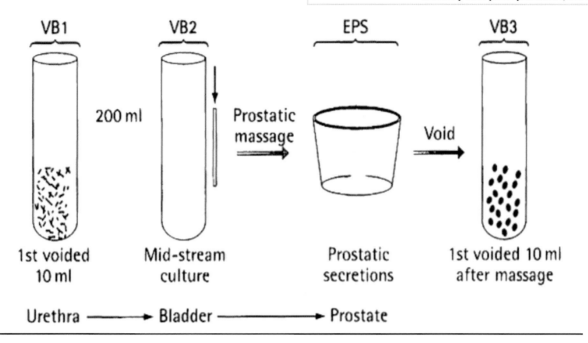

Figure 1. Stamey localisation procedure.

Table 2. Standard uropathogens.

Acknowledged uropathogens – Gram negative
E. Coli
Klebsiella
Pseudomonas

Probable uropathogen – Gram positive
Enterococcus
Staph. aureus

Possible prostate pathogens
Coagulase negative Staphylococcus
Ureaplasma
Anaerobes
Candida
Chlamydia
Trichomonas

Acknowledged non-pathogens
Diphtheroids
Lactobacillus
Corynebacterium

however, have statistically elevated levels of white blood cells in the EPS and VB3 compared to controls [13]. The finding of white blood cells in the EPS of patients with abacterial prostatitis is also episodic in 55% [15]. The method used to detect white cells in the EPS also affects the detection rate of category IIIa compared to IIIb (along with the cut-off used) [16]. The number of leukocytes in EPS does not necessarily correlate with seminal plasma inflammatory cytokines [17]. This is not surprising considering that Krieger found that 39/140 patients with CPPS had "elevated" WBCs in EPS and 40/140 patients had elevated seminal fluid WBCs, while only 10/140 had elevated WBCs in both EPS and seminal fluid [18]. Indeed, patients classified with IIIb prostatitis had higher levels of inflammatory cytokines and evidence of histological inflammation than the control semen specimens, and control subjects' prostate biopsies [19] **(III/B)**. These observations raise intriguing questions. For instance, is the finding of WBCs in the EPS or VB3 of patients with CPPS actually important? Is there such an entity as non-inflammatory CPPS, or has the clinician just assessed the patients at a time when the inflammation is not apparent using the technology available?

The aetiology of chronic prostatitis/ CPPS

The aetiology of chronic prostatitis is not understood. It is however, worth discussing various theories and the evidence for them.

Infection

Conventional micro-organisms are unlikely to cause the symptom complex of chronic prostatitis by themselves. Exhaustive searches for causative pathogenic micro-organisms have been un-rewarding [20, 21]. Weidner reported on 1461 patients, dividing this cohort into four groups (grouped together by their time of presentation to the specialists). This group found that 5%-10% of patients had chronic bacterial prostatitis, similar to the percentage of patients (with symptoms of chronic pelvic pain syndrome) and controls diagnosed with "bacterial prostatitis" by the Stamey localisation [13]. Chlamydia was detected in 14.9% of patients compared to 5% of controls in Weidner's study, which is different to the findings of Doble who studied 50 patients with abacterial prostatitis and found no evidence of chlamydial infection on transperineal prostatic biopsy specimens [22]. Weidner localised Ureaplasma to the prostate in 4%-11% of patients, which is similar to Berger's finding of Ureaplasma in 26% of control subjects [21]. Krieger could find little evidence of infection with conventional uropathogens or possible uropathogens. He reported that 3% of patients had *Chlamydia trachomatis*, 4% had *Mycoplasma genitalium*, 2% had *Trichomonas vaginalis*, and 0% had *Ureaplasma urealyticum* using polymerase chain reaction (PCR) assays to test transperineal prostatic biopsy specimens from 135 patients with chronic idiopathic prostatitis [23]. These studies mentioned, argue against the idea that conventional micro-organisms are causing on-going symptoms in patients with chronic prostatitis **(IIa/B)**.

Cryptic micro-organisms

The role of cryptic organisms will be difficult to assess, as by definition they cannot be cultured by conventional methods. A viral aetiology appears unlikely as Krieger found that none of his 135 patients had CMV or HSV types 1 or 2 [23]. To investigate a microbial cause, investigators have used PCR to amplify microbial 16S ribosomal DNA (rDNA) genes from prostatic biopsies. Krieger demonstrated microbial 16S ribosomal DNA in 77% of the prostates of men with chronic prostatitis but they did not investigate a control group. The presence of 16S rDNA correlated with the finding of EPS leukocytes (p<0.001). Hochreiter found no evidence of 16S ribosomal DNA gene product in the stored prostates of 18 men whose prostates had been preserved at the time of organ donation yet there was no information on whether they had any prostatitis symptoms antemortem [24]. This group of men was much younger that that studied by Krieger (the median age was 26.5). In a subsequent study, Krieger found the 16S ribosomal DNA gene product in 20% of 107 patients with prostate cancer as compared to 46% of 170 men with chronic prostatitis [25]. The median age of the men with prostate cancer was 64 years, and the median age of men with prostatitis was 38 years. These data are difficult to interpret and it is possible that the normal prostate contains a normal flora. It may also be that the men with CPPS have evidence of previous bacterial prostatic infection as DNA is stable. The viability of the micro-organisms is also not certain and efforts to determine the viability of bacteria detected using the broad spectrum 16S ribosomal DNA by using quantitative assays for bacterial mRNA are being investigated [26] **(IIb/B)**.

Dysfunctional high pressure voiding, elevated intraprostatic pressures

Dysfunctional high pressure voiding is also unlikely to be present in significant numbers of patients with chronic prostatitis. Mayo found that only 7/123 patients who attended a specialist chronic pelvic pain clinic had evidence of an abnormal flow rate, defined as a peak flow of under 15ml/sec [27]. Of these seven patients, only two had unequivocal obstruction on video-urodynamics **(III/B)**.

In an interesting study, Mehik has demonstrated elevated intraprostatic pressure in category IIIa compared to category IIIb patients. Both these groups of patients had greater prostatic pressures than control subjects [28]. This group, however, did not control for recent ejaculation and as men with CPPS report reduced libido this may be important [29]. The cause for this elevated intraprostatic pressure is less certain **(IIa/B)**.

Intraprostatic urine reflux

Kirby has demonstrated intraprostatic urine reflux [30]. The ductal anatomy of the prostate makes the peripheral zone ducts more prone to reflux than other areas of the prostate [31]. The existence of urinary reflux is also confirmed by the finding of "secondary" prostatic calculi, which contain urine constituents and uric acid at the core of the stone [32]. The presence of calculi, however, is almost a universal finding on prostatic ultrasound [33]. These calculi are not themselves associated with the symptoms of CPPS and as such it is unlikely that urinary reflux by itself causes CPPS. It is likely, however, that urinary reflux is important in the pathogenesis of acute bacterial prostatitis from a simple urinary tract infection **(III/B)**.

Repetitive perineal trauma

Repetitive perineal trauma is an unlikely cause of CPPS, as there was no association between bicycle riding and a history of prostatitis [1] **(III/B)**.

Abnormal sexual practices

Abnormal sexual patterns are also unlikely to be a cause of CPPS, as a large case controlled study found no differences in the sexual patterns of CPPS patients and asymptomatic age-matched controls [34] **(IIa/B)**.

Interstitial cystitis

Whether interstitial cystitis (IC) is responsible for the symptoms of men diagnosed with CPPS is impossible to say. There are similarities between the two conditions, namely urinary frequency and pelvic pain [35]. There are no gold standard diagnostic tests for either IC or CPPS, so one can only postulate what may be the cause of each. Indeed, it may be that each has a common pathogenesis, namely infection or inflammation starting a subsequent autoimmune process **(IV/C)**.

The autoimmune hypothesis

A number of excellent and largely ignored animal studies demonstrate that it is possible to elicit autoimmune mediated inflammation of the prostate in a rodent [36]. The target auto-antigen appears to be under hormonal control [37, 38]. Human studies demonstrate that some patients with chronic pelvic pain syndrome have auto-reactive T cells to seminal plasma (prostatic) proteins [39, 40]. Cytokine studies point to an inflammatory process of the genital tract and prostate in the group of patients with CPPS compared to controls [41, 42, 43, 44, 45, 46]. The auto-antigen (if indeed present) has not been elucidated. Histological studies suggest a role for CD8+ T cells as the inflammatory grade increases in patients with CPPS [42, 47]. However, the true incidence and pattern of histological inflammation of the prostate of patients with CPPS compared to healthy age-matched controls is not known. In summary, the evidence suggests that it is possible to induce autoimmune mediated inflammation of the male genital tract. The evidence supports the notion that an autoimmune process may be responsible for the symptoms of some (but not necessarily all men) with CPPS. However, conclusive proof of an autoimmune mediated process causing CPPS is not found in the existing medical literature **(IIa/B)**.

The diagnosis and evaluation of men with chronic prostatitis

Chronic prostatitis is a diagnosis of exclusion

The currently accepted evaluation consists of the exclusion of other pathology, which may cause chronic pelvic, perineal, groin, or testicular pain, and urinary symptoms. There are no gold standard diagnostic tests. To this end groin hernia, varicocoele, lower ureteric stones, bladder calculi, bladder malignancy, urethral stricture, bladder outflow obstruction, prostate malignancy, perianal fissures or abscess, interstitial cystitis, Peyronie's disease, and lumbar back pain need to be excluded by careful history, clinical examination, and relevant urine tests.

The National Institutes of Health Chronic Prostatitis Symptom Index Score (CPSI)

This validated symptom score is a useful tool for those managing prostatitis patients (see Table 3). Using 524 men, this questionnaire was developed and validated on three groups of individuals: patients with prostatitis, patients with benign prostatic hyperplasia (BPH), and healthy individuals. An initial questionnaire was produced using focus groups of patients from four tertiary prostatitis centres in the USA to create a draft of 55 questions. This was revised and re-tested to provide a final index of nine questions. These questions outline the experience of chronic prostatitis: location, severity and frequency of genitourinary pain, urinary disturbance and the impact of symptoms on quality of life [48]. It has been assessed for internal consistency, test: re-test reliability, and ability to discriminate between the three groups of men on whom it was validated. It has also been shown to be moderately responsive to change [49] **(IIa/B)**.

The evaluation of men with chronic prostatitis

The Third International Prostatitis Collaborative Network meeting in Washington D.C., USA, held in 2000, proposed guidelines for the evaluation of patients with chronic prostatitis/chronic pelvic pain syndrome. The investigations for CPPS were listed as mandatory, recommended, or optional [50] **(IV/B)**.

Mandatory, recommended and optional investigations

The investigations marked in bold from the list that follows are the investigations this author believes to be the most useful in the evaluation of patients presenting with chronic pelvic pain.

Mandatory investigations include:

- **History.**
- **Physical examination** (including digital rectal examination).
- **Urinalysis/urine culture.**

Recommended evaluations include:

- Lower urinary tract localisation studies.
- **Administering a symptom inventory or index.**
- **Performing a flow rate or residual urine volume estimation.**
- **Obtaining urine for cytological evaluation.**

Optional evaluations include:

- Semen analysis and culture.
- Urethral swab.
- Urodynamics.
- Cystoscopy.
- Transrectal ultrasound of the prostate (TRUS).
- Pelvic imaging studies.
- **Prostate-specific antigen (PSA) determination.**

The mandatory investigations exclude important treatable causes of pelvic pain. The Stamey localisation currently forms the basis of the classification of chronic prostatitis despite the problems discussed previously (the relevance of bacteria in category II patients and the difficulties in separating category IIIa from IIIb). The Stamey localisation should be performed with the foreskin retracted during the procedure and the glans penis cleaned with detergent or an alcohol swab. The prostatic massage may be performed with the patient in the left lateral, or lean over position. Culture medium should be used for normal uropathogens and fastidious micro-organisms. Colony forming unit counts are often much lower than for conventional urine specimens, typically as low as 10^2 CFU/ml. An alternative to the Stamey localisation is the simpler Nickel Pre/Post Massage test [51]. A flow rate helps to exclude urethral stricture disease and bladder outflow obstruction. It is also worthwhile performing urine cytology as Nickel has demonstrated that a relatively small proportion of patients presenting to a specialist clinic (3/150) will have carcinoma *in situ* of the bladder eventually diagnosed [52] **(III/B)**.

Chapter 10

Table 3. NIH Chronic Prostatitis Symptom Index (NIH – CPSI).

Pain or discomfort (circle the appropriate answer)

1. In the last week, have you experienced any pain or
discomfort in the following areas?   **Yes**   **No**
A.   Area between the rectum and the testicles (perineum)   1   0
B.   Testicles   1   0
C.   Tip of the penis (not related to urination)   1   0
D.   Below the waist, in your pubic or bladder area   1   0

2. In the last week, have you experienced: **Yes**   **No**
A.   Pain or burning during urination?   1   0
B.   Pain or discomfort during or after sexual climax (ejaculation)?   1   0

3. How often have you had pain or discomfort in any of these areas over the last week?
Never   0   Rarely   1   Sometimes   2   Often   3   Usually   4   Always   5

4. Which number best describes your average pain or discomfort on the days you had it, over the last week?
0   1   2   3   4   5   6   7   8   9   10
No pain   pain as bad as you can imagine

Urination

5. How often have you had a sensation of not emptying
your bladder completely after you have finished
urinating, over the last week?
Not at all   0
Less than 1 time in 5   1
Less than half the time   2
About half the time   3
More than half the time   4
Almost always   5

6. How often have you had to urinate after finishing urinating,
over the last week?
Not at all   0
Less than 1 time in 5   1
Less than half the time   2
About half the time   3
More than half the time   4
Almost always   5

Impact of symptoms

7. How much have your symptoms kept you from doing
the kinds of things that you would usually do, over the
last week?
None   0
Only a little   1
Some   2
A lot   3

8. How much do you think about your symptoms, over
the last week?
None   0
Only a little   1
Some   2
A lot   3

Quality of life

9. If you are to spend the rest of your life with your symptoms
just the way they have been during the last week, how would
you feel about that?
Delighted   0
Pleased   1
Satisfied   2
Mixed (about equally satisfied and dissatisfied)   3
Mostly dissatisfied   4
Unhappy   5
Terrible   6

Scoring the NIH – Chronic Prostatitis Symptom Index Domains
Pain: total of items 1a, 1b, 1c, 1d, 2a, 2b, 3 and 4   =
Urinary symptoms: total of items 5 and 6   =
Quality of life impact: total of items 7, 8 and 9   =

Checking the patient's serum PSA is useful to exclude the diagnosis of prostate malignancy, as many patients worry that this is the underlying cause of their symptoms [29]. TRUS is less useful, but along with semen analysis may diagnose ejaculatory duct obstruction or Mullerian cyst. Doble has reported on the ultrasound findings of chronic prostatitis and found ultrasonographic signs (high range echoes, mid range echoes, echolucent zones, ejaculatory duct calcification, capsular irregularity, capsular thickness, and peri-urethral abnormalities) associated with chronic abacterial prostatitis [53]. The specificity of these signs, however, limits their utility in the assessment of patients. De la Rosette determined that a normal ultrasound scan could not exclude the diagnosis of non-bacterial prostatitis [33]. Transrectal ultrasound-guided biopsy should only be performed to exclude malignancy in the case of an elevated PSA, unless it is being used to guide prostate biopsy as part of a research study. Semen analysis may be performed for purposes of NIH classification, though studies have shown that men with non-bacterial prostatitis and prostatodynia have semen parameters within the normal range (with the exception of seminal fluid leukocytes) [54, 55, 56, 57]. The semen white count should ideally be performed using a myeloperoxidase, or leukoperoxidase test as differentiation between immature spermatocytes and white cells is impossible using ordinary light microscopy [58, 11] **(IIa/B)**.

A psychological assessment of patients with chronic prostatitis should probably form part of the examination, as authors have all noted depression in patients with chronic prostatitis [59, 60, 61] **(III/B)**.

The treatment of men with chronic prostatitis/ CPPS

Only a few properly conducted randomised placebo-controlled studies (RCT) exist in the literature for chronic prostatitis. This is changing with the NIH funding multicentre North-American randomised controlled trials (RCTs). In spite of these efforts though, there currently remains no gold standard treatment for chronic prostatitis/CPPS.

Alpha-blockers

Alpha-blockers seem to be beneficial in men with category IIIa/IIIb CPPS [62]. In this study, 58 men 55 years and younger were randomised to tamsulosin versus placebo for a period of six weeks with a two-week washout, beforehand. Two visits after randomisation (at two and six weeks) compared the treatment effects. At two weeks there was no statistically significant difference between placebo and tamsulosin, whilst at six weeks tamsulosin was statistically better than placebo with a -3.6 difference in CPSI score (p=0.04). In those patients with severe prostatitis (defined as >75th quartile of the baseline total CPSI score) the difference in treatment was greater, with a CPSI score difference of -8.3 over placebo (p=0.01). This study (and others using alpha-blockers tamsulosin [63], terazosin [64] and alfuzosin [65]) suggests that a longer treatment period (than typically studied for BPH) is required for patients to achieve a relatively modest improvement in symptoms over placebo. Patients who are most symptomatic are likely to gain the greatest benefit **(Ib/A)**.

Antibiotics

Two recently conducted RCTs have studied the role of quinolone antibiotic treatment (levofloxacin [66] and ciprofloxacin [67]) in patients with chronic prostatitis and chronic pelvic pain syndrome. Neither of these studies found any improvement in symptoms in those taking antibiotics over placebo. Antibiotics can no longer be recommended for the treatment of chronic prostatitis on the basis of the best available evidence. This is not surprising when one considers the lack of evidence supporting an infectious aetiology for chronic prostatitis/CPPS **(Ib/A)**.

Anti-inflammatories

Anti-inflammatories have also been studied in two recent RCTs. One studied rofecoxib [68] and the other used naproxen alone and in combination with tamsulosin [63]. Both studies noted a modest (but not statistically significant) improvement in symptoms in those patients taking the anti-inflammatories over placebo. Nickel studied 161 patients and randomised these to placebo, rofecoxib 25mg or rofecoxib 50mg.

He noted that 56% of patients taking 50mg rofecoxib had a >50% reduction in total NIH-CPSI after six weeks of therapy compared to 27% of patients taking placebo. This author studied 83 patients in a pilot study comparing placebo, naproxen 500mg bd, tamsulosin 400mcg od and the combination of tamsulosin and naproxen. At the end of a six-week assessment period it was noted that 18% of patients taking naproxen had a >50% reduction in total NIH-CPSI after six weeks of therapy compared to 5% of patients taking placebo. In this study, the combination of naproxen and tamsulosin was less effective than placebo and was associated with a greater incidence of adverse events [63] **(Ib/A)**.

Hormonal therapy

Finasteride has also been the subject of a multicentre North American placebo-controlled randomised study [69]. In this study, 76 patients were studied for six months. Of the patients treated with finasteride, 75% had at least a 25% improvement in symptoms compared to 54% of the placebo group, whilst 44% of the finasteride group had a >50% improvement in symptoms compared to 27% of the placebo group. These differences did not, however, reach statistical significance **(Ib/A)**.

More recently, mepartricin (which may interfere with the reabsorption of oestrogen from the gut) was studied in category III chronic prostatitis patients [70]. In this small study (26 patients), the total NIH-CPSI decreased from 25 to ten in the mepartricin group and from 25 to 20 in the placebo group after 60 days of treatment. This improvement of symptoms was also associated with a lowering of plasma 17-beta-estradiol in the mepartricin group **(Ib/A)**.

Recommended treatment pathway

Most of the studies quoted in the preceding paragraphs have demonstrated a relatively large placebo effect in patients with chronic prostatitis/ chronic pelvic pain syndrome and the absence of an available cure for the problem. Combined therapies of alpha-blocker and antibiotics [67] and alpha-blockers and anti-inflammatories [64] also seem to lack effect. On the basis of the best available evidence, there are

three levels of treatment for chronic prostatitis recommended **(Ia/A)**:

- The first level includes a sympathetic realistic approach to likely treatment benefit, treatment of depression with referral as appropriate, and allaying fears.
- The second level includes medical options: encouraging study participation, alpha-blockers, anti-inflammatories, amitriptyline, analgesics, finasteride, pentosan polysulfate; non-medical options consisting of pelvic floor relaxation, bladder training, prostatic massage, lifestyle changes, dietary modifications (refer patients to www.prostatitis.org, the web site of the Prostatitis Foundation), donut cushion, psychotherapy, sunlight; and herbal options: quercetin.
- The third level includes transurethral microwave thermotherapy, and pain clinic referral with regional pain blocks.

Conclusions

The evidence presented in this chapter would suggest that the Stamey localisation is likely to fall from use in the determination of "chronic bacterial prostatitis" in those men presenting with symptoms of pelvic pain. Epidemiological studies have shown associations of chronic prostatitis, which should aid in the understanding of aetiology of CPPS, and management of these patients. Case-controlled studies have demonstrated a number of important differences between patients and controls especially seminal plasma cytokine levels and immunology studies. These reports point to an autoimmune process in a substantial number of patients with CPPS, which is precipitated by bacterial genito-urinary infection. Further studies evaluating the immune responses of patients, in particular determining a putative auto-antigen, the role for bacteria in the genesis and continuation of symptoms, and the patients' pain responses to genitourinary insult, should help in our understanding of the pathogenesis of CPPS. Until such time as the aetiology (ies) are fully determined, the diagnosis and treatment remains largely empirical, and currently ineffective.

Chapter 10

Chapter 10

Recommendations   Evidence level

What is the aetiology of chronic prostatitis?

- Unsure but the best available evidence would support a phased pathogenesis   IIa/B
  (that is an infectious phase, an autoimmune phase and a neurogenic-chronic
  pain phase) with potentially multiple entry points to each of these phases.

How do you make the diagnosis?

- This is a diagnosis of exclusion; there are no diagnostic tests which prove the   Ia/A
  entity of chronic prostatitis/chronic pelvic pain syndrome.

How do you evaluate a patient with presumed chronic prostatitis?

- There are a few recommended tests: 1) history, 2) physical examination   IIb/B
  (including digital rectal examination, 3) urinalysis/urine culture, 4)
  administering a symptom inventory or index, 5) performing a flow rate or
  residual urine volume estimation, 6) obtaining urine for cytological
  evaluation and 7) prostate-specific antigen (PSA) determination.

Which treatments work?

- There are no cures yet. Treatments reduce the symptoms slightly. To this end   Ib/A
  alpha-blockers have a role, mepartricin looks interesting but needs further
  evaluation and other treatments (antibiotics, finasteride and anti-
  inflammatories) are even less effective. Analagesics, pelvic floor relaxation
  and pain clinic referral with psychological support are final common
  pathways for those patients who do not spontaneously improve.

References

1. Collins MM, Meigs JB, Barry MJ, *et al.* Prevalence and correlates of prostatitis in the health professionals follow-up study cohort. *J Urol* 2002; 167(3): 1363-6.
2. Mehik A, Hellstrom P, Lukkarinen O, *et al.* Epidemiology of prostatitis in Finnish men: a population-based cross-sectional study *BJU Int* 2000; 86(4): 443-8.
3. Nickel JC, Downey J, Hunter D, Clark J. Prevalence of prostatitis-like symptoms in a population-based study using the National Institutes of Health Chronic Prostatitis Symptom Index. *J Urol* 2001; 165(3): 842-5.
4. Roberts RO, Lieber MM, Rhodes T, Girman CJ, Bostwick DG, Jacobsen SJ. Prevalence of a physician-assigned diagnosis of prostatitis: the Olmsted County Study of Urinary Symptoms and Health Status Among Men. *Urology* 1998; 51(4): 578-84.
5. Wenninger K, Heiman JR, Rothman I, Berghuis JP, Berger RE. Sickness impact of chronic nonbacterial prostatitis and its correlates. *J Urol* 1996; 155(3): 965-8.
6. McNaughton Collins M, MacDonald R, Wilt TJ. Diagnosis and treatment of chronic abacterial prostatitis: a systematic review. *Ann Int Med* 2000; 133(5): 367-81.
7. Nickel JC. *Textbook of Prostatitis.* ISIS, Oxford 1999.
8. Meares EM, Stamey TA. Bacteriologic localization patterns in bacterial prostatitis and urethritis. *Investigative Urology* 1968; 5(5): 492-518.
9. Nickel JC. Prostatitis: evolving management strategies. *Urological Clinics of North America* 1999; 26(4): 737-51.
10. Ludwig M, Schroeder-Printzen I, Ludecke G, Weidner W. Comparison of expressed prostatic secretions with urine after

prostatic massage – a means to diagnose chronic prostatitis/
inflammatory chronic pelvic pain syndrome. *Urology* 2000;
55(2): 175-7.

11. WHO. *Laboratory manual for the examination of human
semen and sperm-cervical mucus interaction.* Cambridge
University Press, Cambridge, 1999.

12. Nickel JC, Downey J, Johnston B, Clark J, Group TC.
Predictors of patient response to antibiotic therapy for the
chronic prostatitis/chronic pelvic pain syndrome: a
prospective multicenter clinical trial. *J Urol* 2001; 165(5):
1539-44.

13. Schaeffer AJ, Knauss JS, Landis JR, *et al.* Leukocyte and
bacterial counts do not correlate with severity of symptoms in
men with chronic prostatitis: the National Institutes of Health
Chronic Prostatitis Cohort Study. *J Urol* 2002; 168(3): 1048-
53.

14. O'Shaughnessy EJ, Parrino PS. Chronic Prostatitis - fact or
fiction? *JAMA* 1956; 160: 540-542.

15. Wright ET, Chmiel JS, Grayhack JT, Schaeffer AJ. Prostatic
fluid inflammation in prostatitis. *J Urol* 1994; 152(6 Pt 2):
2300-3.

16. Muller CH, Berger RE, Mohr LE, Krieger JN. Comparison of
microscopic methods for detecting inflammation in expressed
prostatic secretions. *J Urol 2001*; 166(6): 2518-24.

17. Alexander RB, Ponniah S, Hasday J, Hebel JR. Elevated
levels of proinflammatory cytokines in the semen of patients
with chronic prostatitis/chronic pelvic pain syndrome. *Urology*
1998; 52(5): 744-9.

18. Krieger JN, Jacobs RR, Ross SO. Does the chronic
prostatitis/pelvic pain syndrome differ from nonbacterial
prostatitis and prostatodynia? *J Urol* 2000; 164(5): 1554-8.

19. John H, Barghorn A, Funke G, Sulser T, Hailemariam S, Hauri
D, Joller-Jemelka H. Noninflammatory chronic pelvic pain
syndrome: immunological study in blood, ejaculate and
prostate tissue. *Eur Urol* 2001; 39(1): 72-8.

20. Weidner W, Schiefer HG, Krauss H, Jantos C, Friedrich HJ,
Altmannsberger M. Chronic prostatitis: a thorough search for
etiologically involved microorganisms in 1,461 patients.
Infection 1991; 19(Suppl 3): S119-25.

21. Berger RE, Krieger JN, Kessler D, Ireton RC, Close C,
Holmes KK, Roberts PL. Case-control study of men with
suspected chronic idiopathic prostatitis. *J Urol 1989*; 141(2):
328-31.

22. Doble A, Thomas BJ, Walker MM, Harris JR, Witherow RO,
Taylor-Robinson D. The role of *Chlamydia trachomatis* in
chronic abacterial prostatitis: a study using ultrasound-guided
biopsy. *J Urol* 1989; 141(2): 332-3.

23. Krieger JN, Riley DE, Roberts MC, Berger RE. Prokaryotic
DNA sequences in patients with chronic idiopathic prostatitis.
Journal of Clinical Microbiology 1996; 34(12): 3120-8.

24. Hochreiter WW, Duncan JL, Schaeffer AJ. Evaluation of the
bacterial flora of the prostate using a 16S rRNA gene-based
polymerase chain reaction. *J Urol* 2000; 163(1): 127-30.

25. Krieger JN, Riley DE, Vesella RL, Miner DC, Ross SO, Lange
PH. Bacterial DNA sequences in prostate tissue from patients
with prostate cancer and chronic prostatitis. *J Urol* 2000;
164(4): 1221-8.

26. Krieger JN, Riley DE. Bacteria in the chronic prostatitis-
chronic pelvic pain syndrome: molecular approaches to
critical research questions. *J Urol* 2002; 167(6): 2574-83.

27. Mayo ME, Ross SO, Krieger JN. Few patients with "chronic
prostatitis" have significant bladder outlet obstruction.
Urology 1998; 52(3): 417-21.

28. Mehik A, Hellstrom P, Nickel JC, Kilponen A, Leskinen M,
Sarpola A, Lukkarinen O. The chronic prostatitis-chronic
pelvic pain syndrome can be characterized by prostatic tissue
pressure measurements. *J Urol* 2002; 167(1): 137-40.

29. Mehik A, Hellstrom P, Sarpola A, Lukkarinen O, Jarvelin MR.
Fears, sexual disturbances and personality features in men
with prostatitis: a population-based cross-sectional study in
Finland. *BJU Int* 2001; 88(1): 35-8.

30. Kirby RS, Lowe D, Bultitude MI, Shuttleworth KE. Intraprostatic urinary reflux: an aetiological factor in abacterial
prostatitis. *Br J Urol* 1982; 54(6): 729-31.

31. Blacklock NJ. Anatomical factors in prostatitis. *Br J Urol*
1974; 46(1): 47-54.

32. Torres Ramirez C, Aguilar Ruiz J, Zuluaga Gomez A, Espuela
Orgaz, R, Del Rio Samper S. A crystallographic study of
prostatic calculi. *J Urol* 1980; 124(6): 840-3.

33. de la Rosette JJ, Karthaus HF, Debruyne FM.
Ultrasonographic findings in patients with nonbacterial
prostatitis. *Urol Int* 1992; 48(3): 323-6.

34. Pontari MA, Litwin MS, O'Leary MP, McNaughton Collins M,
Calhoun E, Knauss, J, Landis JR. A case-controlled study of
epidemiologic factors in men with chronic pelvic pain
syndrome. *J Urol* 2002; 167 (suppl): 24-25.

35. Kusek JW, Nyberg LM. The epidemiology of interstitial
cystitis: is it time to expand our definition? *Urology* 2001; 57(6
Suppl 1): 95-9.

36. Taguchi O, Kojima A, Nishizuka Y. Experimental autoimmune
prostatitis after neonatal thymectomy in the mouse. *Clinical
and Experimental Immunology* 1985; 60(1): 123.

37. Taguchi O, Nishizuka Y. Self tolerance and localized
autoimmunity. Mouse models of autoimmune disease that
suggest tissue-specific suppressor T cells are involved in self
tolerance. *The Journal of Experimental Medicine* 1987;
165(1): 146-56.

38. Taguchi O, Kontani K, Ikeda H, Kezuka T, Takeuchi M,
Takahashi T. Tissue-specific suppressor T cells involved in
self-tolerance are activated extrathymically by self-antigens.
Immunology 1994; 82(3): 365-9.

39. Alexander RB, Brady F, Ponniah S. Autoimmune prostatitis:
evidence of T cell reactivity with normal prostatic proteins.
Urology 1997; 50(6): 893-9.

40. Batstone GRD, Doble A, Gaston JSH. Autoimmune T cell
responses to seminal plasma in chronic pelvic pain syndrome
(CPPS). *Clinical and Experimental Immunology* 2002; 128:
302-307.

41. Alexander RB, Ponniah S, Hasday J, Hebel JR. Elevated
levels of proinflammatory cytokines in the semen of patients
with chronic prostatitis/chronic pelvic pain syndrome. *Urology*
1998; 52(5): 744-9.

42. John H, Barghorn A, Funke G, Sulser T, Hailemariam S, Hauri
D, Joller-Jemelka H. Noninflammatory chronic pelvic pain

syndrome: immunological study in blood, ejaculate and prostate tissue. *Eur Urol* 2001; 39(1): 72-8.

43. Miller LJ, Fischer KA, Goralnick SJ, Litt M, Burleson JA, Albertsen P, Kreutzer DL. Interleukin-10 levels in seminal plasma: implications for chronic prostatitis-chronic pelvic pain syndrome. *J Urol* 2002; 167(2 Pt 1): 753-6.

44. Miller LJ, Fischer KA, Goralnick SJ, Litt M, Burleson JA, Albertsen P, Kreutzer DL. Nerve growth factor and chronic prostatitis/chronic pelvic pain syndrome. *Urology* 2002; 59(4): 603-8.

45. Orhan I, Onur R, Ilhan N, Ardicoglu A. Seminal plasma cytokine levels in the diagnosis of chronic pelvic pain syndrome. *Int J Urol* 2001; 8(9): 495-9.

46. Hochreiter WW, Nadler RB, Koch AE, Campbell PL, Ludwig M, Weidner W, Schaeffer AJ. Evaluation of the cytokines interleukin 8 and epithelial neutrophil activating peptide 78 as indicators of inflammation in prostatic secretions. *Urology* 2000; 56(6): 1025-9.

47. Doble A. *Textbook of Prostatitis*. ISIS, Oxford, 1999.

48. Litwin MS, McNaughton-Collins M, Fowler FJ, Nickel JC, Calhoun EA, Pontari MA, Alexander RB, Farrar JT, O'Leary MP. The National Institutes of Health Chronic Prostatitis Symptom Index: development and validation of a new outcome measure. Chronic Prostatitis Collaborative Research Network. *J Urol* 1999; 162(2): 369-75.

49. Turner JA, Ciol MA, Von Korff M, Berger R. Validity and responsiveness of the National Institutes of Health Chronic Prostatitis Symptom Index. *J Urol* 2003; 69(2): 580-3.

50. Nickel JC. Clinical evaluation of the man with chronic prostatitis/chronic pelvic pain syndrome. *Urology* 2002; 60: 20-23.

51. Nickel JC. The Pre and Post Massage Test (PPMT): a simple screen for prostatitis. *Tech Urology* 1997; 3(1): 38-43.

52. Nickel JC, Arden D, Downey J. Cytologic evaluation of urine is important in evaluation of chronic prostatitis. *Urology* 2002; 60(2): 225-7.

53. Doble A, Carter SS. Ultrasonographic findings in prostatitis. *Urological Clinics of North America*, 1989; 16(4): 763-72.

54. Christiansen E, Tollefsrud A, Purvis K. Sperm quality in men with chronic abacterial prostatovesiculitis verified by rectal ultrasonography. *Urology* 1991; 38(6): 545-9.

55. Weidner W, Jantos C, Schiefer HG, Haidl G, Friedrich HJ. Semen parameters in men with and without proven chronic prostatitis. *Archives of Andrology* 1991; 26(3): 173-83.

56. Leib Z, Bartoov B, Eltes F, Servadio C. Reduced semen quality caused by chronic abacterial prostatitis: an enigma or reality? *Fertility and Sterility* 1994; 61(6): 1109-16.

57. Krieger JN, Berger RE, Ross SO, Rothman I, Muller CH. Seminal fluid findings in men with nonbacterial prostatitis and prostatodynia. *Journal of Andrology* 1996; 17(3): 310-8.

58. Wolff H. The biologic significance of white blood cells in semen. *Fertility and Sterility* 1995; 63(6): 1143-57.

59. de la Rosette JJ, Ruijgrok MC, Jeuken JM, Karthaus HF, Debruyne FM. Personality variables involved in chronic prostatitis. *Urology* 1993; 42(6): 654-62.

60. Berghuis JP, Heiman JR, Rothman I, Berger RE. Psychological and physical factors involved in chronic idiopathic prostatitis. *J Psychosom Res* 1996; 41(4): 313-25.

61. Egan KJ, Krieger JN. Psychological problems in chronic prostatitis patients with pain. *Clinical Journal of Pain* 1994; 10(3): 218-26.

62. Nickel JC, Narayan P, McKay J, Doyle C. Treatment of chronic prostatitis/chronic pelvic pain syndrome with tamsulosin: a randomised double blind trial. *J Urol* 2004; 171(4): 1594-7.

63. Batstone GRD, Lynch J, Doble A. A randomised-placebo controlled pilot study of tamsulosin, naproxen, and combination in category IIIa/IIIb chronic prostatitis/chronic pelvic pain syndrome (CPPS). *BJU Int* 2004; 93(S4): 105.

64. Cheah PY, Liong ML, Yuen KH, The CL, Khor T, Yang JR, Yap HW, Krieger JN. Terazosin therapy for chronic prostatitis/chronic pelvic pain syndrome: a randomised, placebo controlled trial. *J Urol* 2003; 69(2): 592-6.

65. Mehik A, Alas P, Nickel JC, Sarpola A, Helstrom PJ. Alfuzosin treatment for chronic prostatitis/chronic pelvic pain syndrome: a prospective, randomised, double-blind, placebo-controlled, pilot study. *Urology* 2003; 62(2): 425-9.

66. Nickel JC, Downey J, Clark J, Casey RW, Pommerville PJ, Barkin J, Steinhoff G, Brock G, Patrick AB, Flax S, Goldfarb B, Palmer BW, Zadra J. Levofloxacin for chronic prostatitis/chronic pelvic pain syndrome in men: a randomised placebo-controlled multicenter trial. *Urology* 2003; 62(4): 614-7.

67. Alexander RB, Propert KJ, *et al*. A randomized trial of Ciprofloxacin and Tamsulosin in men with chronic prostatitis/chronic pelvic pain syndrome. *J Urol* 2004; 171(4) Supplement: 61.

68. Nickel JC, Pontari M, Moon T, Gittleman M, Malek G, Farrington J, Pearson J, Krupa D, Bach M, Drisko J. A randomized placebo controlled multicenter study to evaluate the safety and efficacy of rofecoxib in the treatment of chronic nonbacterial prostatitis. *J Urol* 2003; 169(4): 1401-5.

69. Nickel JC, Downey J, Pontari MA, *et al*. A randomized placebo-controlled multicentre study to evaluate the safety and efficacy of finasteride for male chronic pelvic pain syndrome (category IIIA chronic nonbacterial prostatitis). *BJU Int* 2004; 93(7): 991-5.

70. De Rose AF, Gallo F, Giglio M, Carmignani G. Role of mepartricin in category III chronic nonbacterial prostatitis/chronic pelvic pain syndrome: a randomised propective placebo-controlled trial. *Urology* 2004; 63(1): 13-16.

Chapter 11

Lower urinary tract symptoms suggestive of benign prostatic hyperplasia: what is the evidence for rational diagnosis?

Andrea Tubaro MD FEBU

Associate Professor of Urology

Cosimo De Nunzio MD

Consultant Urologist

Alberto Trucchi MD FEBU

Assistant Professor of Urology

SANT' ANDREA HOSPITAL, ROME, ITALY

Introduction

An enlarged prostatic gland is one of the most common diagnoses in older men and is due to a histopathological condition called "benign prostatic hyperplasia" (BPH) which usually develops after the fourth decade of life. Clinical manifestations of BPH include symptoms, signs and sequelae of urinary obstruction caused by the enlarged prostate. Although not life-threatening, clinical manifestations of lower urinary tract symptoms (LUTS) affect between 15% and 30% of men aged over 60 years and patients seek treatment to improve their quality of life. Some men are asymptomatic but might still be obstructed if appropriately investigated [1,2] **(I/A, IV/C)**. An accurate assessment of patients with BPH has to consider the possible relationship between benign prostatic enlargement, lower urinary tract symptoms (LUTS) and signs of bladder outlet obstruction, to quantify the severity of benign prostatic enlargement (BPE) related symptoms and signs, and to rule out the presence of cancer. The 5th International Consultation on BPH summarised the current understanding of the disease and outlined the definition of recommended and optional diagnostic tests that should be used in the assessment of BPH. Recommended tests to be performed in all patients with LUTS and BPE include: medical history, quantification of symptoms and bother, physical examination, urinalysis, prostate specific antigen (PSA) and frequency volume chart. Optional tests include: uroflometry, post-void residual volume, upper urinary tract imaging, pressure-flow studies, transrectal ultrasound (TRUS), upper tract imaging by ultrasonography or intravenous urography and endoscopy of the lower urinary tract. These recommendations are based on a thorough review of the available literature and the opinion of recognised experts [3] **(IV/C)**. Numerous other national and international guidelines are available: their recommendations may differ because of variation in experts' opinion, national health system resources, reimbursement issues, etc. So far in clinical practice, the management of LUTS is still based on the physician and the patient's shared decision-making and to recommendations existing in individual countries on BPH management [4] **(IV/C)**.

Methodology

In this chapter, based on a Medline, EMBASA literature search (search term "BPH investigations and diagnosis", limited to Human/English language/review articles/publication), we have captured all published data covering the period from 1998 to August 2003 regarding investigations of BPH. A total of 300 abstracts were listed, 100 full text papers were reviewed and 32 were considered of interest to define the evidence on BPH diagnosis.

Medical history and general physical examination

Not all guidelines have discussed the importance of a medical history in the diagnosis of BPH. The American Urological Association (AUA) [5] **(IV/C)** and the 5th International Consultation on BPH [4] highly recommended that a detailed medical history is taken focusing on the urinary tract to identify other causes of voiding dysfunction or comorbidities that may complicate treatment or may necessitate more accurate diagnostic tools. A general physical examination with specific attention to the presence or absence of a distended bladder, excoriation of the genitals secondary to urinary incontinence, evidence of urethral discharge and a focused neurological examination is also highly recommended. The presence of cancer should also be excluded by digital rectal examination (DRE). However, the specificity and sensitivity of DRE for prostatic cancer detection is low [6] **(III/B)**; DRE also underestimates the prostatic volume as compared with transrectal ultrasound or magnetic resonance [7] **(III/B)**.

Assessment of lower urinary tract symptoms and quality of life

The first step in the evaluation of men with LUTS suggestive of BPH should include careful assessment of the patient's symptoms. Symptoms suggestive of BPH are generally difficult to quantify and analyse and they can be divided into voiding and storage symptoms. These symptoms can be associated with bladder outlet obstruction (BOO) due to BPH or may occur in the absence of BOO but are commonly seen in patients with impaired detrusor contractility or as a result of detrusor overactivity. Most patients seek treatments for BPH because LUTS affect their quality of life. Symptom quantification is of importance to

evaluate the severity of the disease and the response to treatment. Different urinary tract symptom questionnaires are available in the literature. Questionnaires may be self-administered or filled by an interviewer; they must be reliable, responsive and validated. Initial symptom assessment instruments were the Boyarsky [8] **(IV/C)** and Madsen Iverson [9] **(IV/C)** scores developed in the late 1970s and early 1980s. They were used in numerous reports but there is no evidence of their reliability and validity. The American Urological Association questionnaire described by Barry and his colleagues [10] **(IV/C)** in the early 1990s has been adopted by the International Consultation on BPH as the International Prostatic Symptom Score (IPSS) and has become the international standard. The correlation of IPSS and other variables such as prostate volume, urinary flow rate, post-void residual urine and BOO is known to be low, but different studies have shown its validity as an outcome measure [11-12] **(IV/C, III/B)**.

The International Continence Society (ICS) introduced its own questionnaire to measure levels of urinary symptoms in middle-aged and elderly men. The ICS-BPH questionnaire is completed by the patient and contains questions on symptoms, bothersomeness, quality of life and sexual function. The ICS-BPH questionnaire has a high level of validity and reliability; it revealed a lower incidence of storage symptoms compared with the IPSS questionnaire [13] **(II/B)**. Terminal dribble which was not considered in the IPSS questionnaire was frequently reported in the ICS form [14] **(I/A)**. However, the Committee for the initial evaluation of LUTS at the 5th International Consultation on BPH [15] **(IV/C)** still recommends IPSS with the Quality of Life (QoL) question as the standard questionnaire in patients with BPH. Most men seek treatment for BPH because of the bothersome nature of their symptoms which affect the quality of their life. QoL questionnaires can be generic or disease-specific; a number of instruments have been made available over the years. One of the best known generic tools is the medical outcomes study 36-item short form healthy survey (SF36). Using this score Hunter et al [16] **(I/A)** observed that 9%-49% of men with moderate or severe urinary symptoms reported interference with some of their daily activities and that increasing symptom severity was associated with worsening quality of life. More conventional disease-specific tools to evaluate the impact of LUTS on quality of life include:

- The ICS male questionnaire and the Danish Prostatic symptom score, which measure symptom severity and frequency.
- The BPH Impact Index, which measures the impact of symptoms on daily activities.
- The Disease Specific Quality of Life question of the IPSS which measures quality of life as it is impacted and impaired by BPH and which is still considered as a standard by the International Consultation on BPH [5,15].

Serum creatinine and urinalysis

Serum creatinine evaluation is recommended by several BPH guidelines [4]. However, there is no evidence on its utility in the first-line evaluation of men with LUTS related to BPH. Renal insufficiency appears to be no more common in men with BPH than in men of the same age group in the general population [5]. In several large clinical BPH trials, renal failure has been reported in less than 1% of the population evaluated [5].

Urinalysis is considered an inexpensive test which does not require sophisticated technologies and is generally recommended by almost all BPH guidelines. Since LUTS is frequently associated with urinary tract infection, bladder carcinoma, distal ureteral or bladder stones, microscopic examination of the urine sediment helps in the differential diagnosis of these conditions [15].

Prostate specific antigen

Screening for prostatic cancer is one reason why men over 50 will consult their family doctor or a urology clinic. Prostate Specific Antigen (PSA) has been primarily used in the diagnosis and treatment of prostatic cancer since its introduction in the 1980s; however, it is also produced by benign prostatic epithelial cells and many patients with BPH and LUTS might have a raised PSA. So far, an evaluation of PSA in the adult male population is no longer limited to the diagnosis of prostatic cancer, but has also found a

role in the management of patients with BPH. Serum PSA proved to be a surrogate of prostate volume, and has been shown to be a strong predictor of the risk of acute urinary retention and the need for surgery in men with BPH [17] (I/A). The Longitudinal Baltimore Study of Aging also showed evidence for a clear increase in the risk of prostate enlargement in each cohort (from 40 to 69.9 years) for higher values of serum PSA levels [18] (I/B). However, the routine use of PSA serum analysis for screening prostatic cancer is still debated. The European Urology Association [19] (IV/C), and the American Urological Association guidelines [5] on BPH suggest that the benefit and risks of PSA testing should be discussed with the patient. PSA testing is recommended in men with LUTS and life expectancy of over ten years in whom the diagnosis of prostate cancer would change the management of the patient's voiding symptoms. The Committee on initial evaluation of LUTS of the 5th International Consultation on BPH also support this practice [15].

Frequency volume chart (voiding diary)

Voiding charts are simple to complete and can provide useful clinical information: they are considered by the 5th Consultation on BPH [3] as a mandatory test in the initial evaluation of men with LUTS. The voiding charts give evidence of frequency, mean volume voided, nocturia, urge, urge incontinence and 24-hour urine volume. Voiding diaries are particularly used in patients with nocturia as the dominant symptom. A voiding diary filled out for at least one 24-hour period should help to distinguish between patients with nocturia, nocturnal polyuria or excessive fluid intake. The frequency volume chart allows the investigator to compare the patient's mean voided volume at home and the urinary volume assessed by uroflowmetry in the urodynamic lab [20] (IV/C).

Post-void residual (PVR) urine

The 5th International Consultation on BPH considered the evaluation of post-void residual urine a useful but optional test in the initial diagnostic assessment of patients with LUTS related to BPH [3]. It should be calculated by measurement of bladder height, width and length obtained by transabdominal ultrasonography [21] (IV/C). However, because of the marked variability of residual urine volume, the test should be repeated whenever significant volumes are measured which might suggest a change in the treatment plan [20]. Large PVR volumes may indicate bladder dysfunction and predict a poor response to treatment and in particular, to watchful waiting strategies. Because of large patient variability it is not possible to establish a PVR cut-off point for decision-making. The value of 50-100ml has been considered as a possible lower threshold to define abnormal residual urine [5]. Although high residual urine volumes have been linked to urinary tract infection and renal failure in paediatric and neurogenic populations, there is no evidence of a higher incidence of urinary tract infection, renal failure, or bothersome symptoms in adult male patients with large amounts of residual urine [22] (III/B). So far, no level of residual urine mandates invasive therapy [5]. However, several national guidelines still consider PVR evaluation as a recommended test in the evaluation of men with BPH [4].

Urodynamic assessment

The role of urodynamics in the management of patients with LUTS related to BPH is still an unresolved issue. Analysis of the peer-reviewed literature showed many reasons to support the use of uroflow and pressure-flow studies in BPH patients, although evidence for making the latter test mandatory is still weak.

The uroflow study is the most commonly performed urodynamic test, although it is unable to discriminate BOO from detrusor underactivity. Uroflometry is recommended as a diagnostic test in the initial work-up of patients with LUTS by several national guidelines on BPH [4], but it is considered an optional test by the 5th International Consultation on BPH [20]. It is a simple, non-invasive test that can identify patients with an abnormal voiding pattern and monitor changes in voiding dynamics over time in watchful waiting programmes and follow-up of medical therapy,

physical treatment or surgical therapies. The prognostic ability of maximum free flow rate (PFR) in the diagnosis of bladder outlet obstruction is known to be in the following range [20]:

Peak flow (QMax)	Probability of obstruction
Less than 10ml/s	90%
10-14ml/s	67%
15ml/s or more	30%

Uroflow studies are limited by inter-test variability over repeated tests, related to the patient's learning effect, circadian effect, uroflometer artefacts and intra-observer, inter-observer variation from manual correction of uroflow traces. Rowan et al [23] (IV/C) showed artefacts (particularly spikes) in up to 20% of flow traces: the computer may fail to recognise these artefacts thereby printing a false reading of Qmax. So, the investigator should manually check and correct each flow for artefacts rather than accept the output from the computer uroflometer. There is also evidence that a single flow rate should not be considered as adequate. Repeated flow measurements in the same patients after two weeks showed a significant variability in normal recorded measurements including the Qmax with a mean difference of 0.1ml/sec but a standard deviation of 3.2ml/sec [24] (III/B). So far, there is widespread evidence that a single urine flow measurement is unsatisfactory and three flow measurements should be performed in a urine flow clinic as a vital part of the patient's assessment [20].

Pressure flow studies are considered an optional test by several international guidelines [20]. However, bladder outlet obstruction can only be diagnosed by urodynamic assessment of voiding pressure and flow. The rationale for using pressure flow studies in the evaluation of men with LUTS related to BPH derives from the lack of correlation between symptoms, an enlarged prostate gland, and the presence of BOO. So far, the urodynamic Committee of the 5th International Consultation on BPH [20] stated that pressure flow studies remain the only means of establishing the presence of BOO. They also recommend their use in all patients before surgery, particularly in patients with a PFR >10ml/sec and whenever the patient's history does not agree with

Lower urinary tract symptoms suggestive of benign prostatic hyperplasia: what is the evidence for rational diagnosis?

Chapter 11

clinical findings [20]. Although different nomograms exist to assess BOO status, the ICS nomograms should be used as the method of choice to define patients as obstructed, non-obstructed or equivocal. There is also some evidence in the literature that the outcome of surgery may be better in men with obstruction than in those who are not obstructed as defined by pre-operative pressure flow studies [25] **(III/B)**. Jensen *et al* [26] **(III/B)** observed that a subjective unsatisfactory outcome after TURP was 7% in urodynamically obstructed patients and 22% in unobstructed patients. Rodrigues *et al* also [27] **(III/B)** observed that urodynamic studies provide great predictive value of clinical improvement after prostatic relief but they also properly predict the poor clinical results in non-obstructed patients. According to AUA guidelines on BPH [5], pressure flow studies should also be considered a mandatory test in men with LUTS who have failed previous invasive therapy or who have concomitant neurological disease known to affect bladder function, or in men in whom the physician believes that the study outcome would change the management strategy [5].

Imaging of the urinary tract

Imaging of the upper and lower urinary tract has been used for several years as part of the diagnostic assessment of men with LUTS related to BPH [28]. Nowadays, the routine use of upper urinary tract imaging by means of intravenous urography or renal ultrasound is not recommended in most guidelines on BPH management. Many urologists do not take images of the upper urinary tract routinely because tumours and kidney stones or failure are not more frequent in men with LUTS related to BPH than in healthy men [2]. However, renal ultrasound should be considered as the imaging modality of the upper urinary tract in patients with BPH and a history of urinary tract infection, urolithiasis, haematuria or renal insufficiency [4]. Lower urinary tract imaging should be performed to assess prostate size and shape, asymptomatic bladder neoplasms, diverticula, stones and wall thickness. Prostate volume can be estimated by the suprapubic route with sufficient accuracy. The advantage of transrectal versus suprapubic ultrasound (TRUS) imaging is the possibility of evaluating prostate morphology and transition zone index (TZI). Choi *et al* [29] **(I/A)** showed a higher mean TZI value and IPSS value in Korean men compared with Caucasian and Hispanic cohorts; they confirmed a relationship between TZI and LUTS and suggested the possible relationship between the higher TZI observed in Korean men (despite a lower mean prostate volume) and the greater severity of LUTS in this population.

At this time there is no evidence to consider TRUS as a valuable tool for detecting early prostatic cancer or to excluding prostate cancer in men presenting with LUTS. However, it should be used to guide accurate needle placement during transrectal prostatic biopsy [30] **(IV/C)**. Currently, prostate ultrasound (transrectal or transabdominal) should be considered as an optional test in the management of patients with BPH. It may be an appropriate test when minimally invasive therapy or surgical operations are considered. The size and shape of the prostate and the presence of an intravesical lobe clearly seen on ultrasound should be considered in selecting patients for transurethral microwave heat treatment (TUNA) or other minimally invasive therapies as well as for the selection of transurethral prostatic incision (TUIP) versus transurethral prostatic resection (TURP) [5]. Magnetic resonance imaging or computer tomographic images are an alternative method for lower urinary tract imaging with somewhat greater precision in the estimation of prostate volume than transrectal or transabdominal ultrasonography, but their higher cost and lower availability limit their usefulness to clinical research [31] **(IV/C)**.

Endoscopy

Urethrocystoscopy is the standard endoscopic procedure to evaluate the lower urinary tract. It can provide information about prostate size, cause and severity of BOO, about the presence of bladder diverticula, trabeculation or stones, about bladder neck anatomy and the presence of urethral stones or diverticula. Because of the low prognostic value of bladder endoscopy for the diagnosis of BOO, the test remains optional in all the guidelines considered [32] **(III/B)**. So far, this test should not be used in the initial evaluation of patients with LUTS but is appropriate in men with a history of microscopic or gross haematuria, urethral stricture, bladder cancer, or prior lower urinary tract surgery. It should not be performed whenever watchful waiting or medical therapy has been proposed as the treatment of choice and it remains optional in patients scheduled for surgery [5].

Conclusions

Analysis of the different guidelines for the management of patients with LUTS due to BPH show that most recommendations are based on low grade evidence and sometimes only on experts' opinion. Table 1 summarises a possible list of recommended and optional tests derived from all available guidelines.

The major findings of this review are shown in Table 1. Although evidence is lacking for a number of points there is evidence to support some arguments. In the initial evaluation of men with LUTS, the 5th Consultation

on BPH and several national and international guidelines consider the following as mandatory diagnostic steps: a full medical history with evaluation of LUTS with a symptom questionnaire and the bother score, a physical examination including a digital rectal examination, urinalysis, serum prostate specific antigen and urinary flow charts. Optional tests to be used at the urologist's discretion comprise: creatinine levels, renal ultrasound, urodynamic evaluation, post-void residual urine, transrectal ultrasound, lower urinary tract imaging and endoscopy. Several national guidelines, on the basis of local clinical practice, recommend some of these optional tests in the initial evaluation process of patients with LUTS. However, there is no evidence to consider them mandatory at the initial evaluation process.

In the readers' interest, we strongly suggest that all published guidelines should provide the grade of evidence upon which the recommendations are based. The benefit of such a policy is two-fold as it provides substantiation to the suggested guiding principles and identifies areas for future research.

Table 1. Diagnostic evaluation of men with LUTS.

Initial evaluation: recommended tests

- Medical history
- Quantification of symptoms by means of the International Symptom Score with Bother Score
- Physical digital rectal examination
- Urinalysis
- Frequency-volume chart (voiding diary)
- Serum Prostate Specific Antigen

Urologic evaluation: optional tests

- Uroflowmetry
- Post-void residual urine
- Serum creatinine
- Pressure-flow studies
- Imaging of the prostate by means of transrectal or transabdominal ultrasound
- Imaging of the upper urinary tract by means of renal ultrasound or intravenous urography
- Urethrocystoscopy

Recommendations	Evidence level

Is any investigation needed at all in patients referred for LUTS and benign prostatic enlargement?

◆ Yes, because a causative relation between LUTS and BPE needs to be established and other possible causes of LUTS (eg. urinary tract infection, bladder neoplasms or stones) must be ruled out.	IV/C

Which are the mandatory examinations to be performed in all patients before any medical treatment is initiated?

◆ Medical history.	IV/C
◆ Physical examination including DRE.	III/B
◆ Assessment of LUTS severity and bothersomeness.	IV/C
◆ Frequency volume chart.	IV/C
◆ Urinalysis.	IV/C
◆ Serum creatinine.	IV/C
◆ PSA.	IV/C
◆ Post-void residual urine.	IV/C

Which are the optional tests to be performed in selected patients, in patients who do not respond to treatment and eventually before minimally invasive treatment or surgery?

◆ Uroflowmetry.	III/B
◆ Pressure flow study.	III/B
◆ Ultrasound imaging of the bladder and prostate.	IV/C
◆ Endoscopy.	IV/C

Areas for future research

- Clinical outcome of patients with or without detrusor instability.
- Clinical outcome of patients with or without detrusor underactivity.
- The prognostic value of detrusor hypertrophy for the clinical outcome of medical and surgical treatment of BPH.
- The prognostic value of prostate morphology (eg. elevated bladder neck, middle lobe) and volume for the clinical outcome of medical and surgical treatment of BPH.
- The prognostic value of post-void residual urine volume for complications of BPH (eg. urinary tract infection and renal failure).

Chapter 11

Chapter 11

References

1. Emberton M, Andriole GL, De La Rosette J, *et al*. Benign prostatic hyperplasia: a progressive disease of aging men. *Urology* 2003; 61: 267-273.

2. Thorpe A, Neal D. Benign Prostatic Hyperplasia. *The Lancet* 2003; 361: 1359-67.

3. Chatelain C, Denis L, Foo JKT, *et al*. Evaluation and treatment of Lower Urinary Tract Symptoms (LUTS) in older men. In: *Benign Prostatic Hyperplasia*. C Chatelain, L Denis, Foo KT *et al*, Eds. June 25-28, 2000. Health Publication Ltd, Paris, Plymouth, UK, 2001: 519-534.

4. Roehrborn CG, Bartsch G, Kirby R, *et al*. Guidelines for the diagnosis and treatment of benign prostatic hyperplasia: a comparative international overview. *Urology* 2001; 58: 642-650.

5. AUA guidelines on management of benign prostatic hyperplasia (2003). Chapter 1: diagnosis and treatment recommendation. *J Urol* 2003; 170: 530-547.

6. Chodak GW, Kotler P, Shoenberg H. Routine screening for prostate cancer using the digital rectal examination. *Prog Clin Biol Res* 1988; 269-87.

7. Roehrborn CG, Sech S, Montoya J, Rhodes T, Girman CJ. Interexaminer reliability and validity of three dimensional model to assess prostate volume by digital rectal examination. *Urology* 2001; 57: 1087.

8. Boyarsky S, Jones G, Paulson DF, *et al*. A new look at bladder neck obstruction by the Food and Drug Administration: guidelines for investigation of benign prostatic hypertrophy. *Trans Am Assoc Genitourinary Surg* 1977; 68: 29-36.

9. Madsen PO, Iversen P. A point for selecting operative candidates. In: *Benign Prostatic Hypertrophy*. Hinman F, Jr Ed. Springer Verlag, New York, 1983: 763-65.

10. Barry MJ, Fowler FJ Jr, O'Leary MP, Bruskewitz RC, Holtgrewe HL, Mebust WK, Cocket AT. The American Urological Association symptom index for benign prostatic hyperplasia. The Measurement Committee of the American Urological Association. *J Urol* 1992; 148(5): 1549-57.

11. Barry M. Evaluation of symptoms and quality of life in men with benign prostatic hyperplasia. *Urology* 2001; 58: 25-32.

12. Sirls LT, Kirkemo AK, Jay J. Lack of correlation of the AUA symptom/index with urodynamic bladder outlet obstruction. *Neurourol* 1996; 15: 447-457.

13. Donovan JL, Abrams P, Peters TJ, *et al*. The ICS BPH study: the psychometric validity and reliability of ICS/male questionnaire. *Br J Urol* 1996; 77: 554-562.

14. Bertaccini A, Vassallo F, Martino F, *et al*. Symptoms, bothersomeness and quality of life in patients with LUTS suggestive of BPH. *Eur Urol* 2001; 40: 13-18.

15. Resnick M, Ackermann R, Bosch J, *et al*. Initial evaluation of LUTS. In: *Benign Prostatic Hyperplasia*. Chatelain C, Denis L, Foo KT, *et al*, Eds. June 25-28, 2000. Health Publication Ltd, Plymouth, UK, 2001: 169-202.

16. Hunter DJW, McKee M, Black NA, Sanderson CFB, *et al*. Health status and quality of life of British men with lower urinary tract symptoms: results from the SF36. *Urology* 1995; 45: 962-71.

17. Roehrborn CG, Malice M, cook TJ and Girman CJ. Clinical predictors of spontaneous acute urinary retention in men with LUTS and clinical BPH: a comprehensive analysis of the pooled placebo groups of several large clinical Trials. *Urology* 2001; 58: 210.

18. Wright EJ, Fang J, Metter EJ, *et al*. Prostate specific antigen predicts the long-term risk of prostate enlargement: results from the Baltimore longitudinal study of Aging. *J Urol* 2002; 167: 2484-88.

19. De L Rosette JJMCH, Alivizatos G, Madersbaacher S, Perchino M, Thomas D, *et al*. EAU guidelines on benign prostatic hyperplasia. *Eur Urol* 2001; 40: 256-263.

20. Abrams P, Griffiths D, Hofner K, Liao L, Schafer W, Tubaro A, Zimmern P. In: *Benign Prostatic Hyperplasia*. Chatelain C, Denis L, Foo KT, *et al*, Eds. June 25-28, 2000. Health Publication Ltd, Plymouth, UK, 2001: 227-281.

21. Griffiths D, Hofner K, van Mastrigt R, *et al*. Standardization of terminology of lower urinary tract function: Pressure flow studies of voiding urethral resistance and urethral obstruction. *Neurourol Urodyn* 1997; 16: 1-18.

22. Merritt JL. Residual urine volume: correlate of urinary tract infection in patients with spinal cord injury. *Arch Phys Med Rehabil* 1981; 62(11): 558-61.

23. Rowan D, James ED, Kramer AE, *et al*. Urodynamic equipment: technical aspects. Produced by the International Continence Society Working Party on Urodynamic Equipment. *J Med Eng Technol* 1987; 11(2): 57-64.

24. Reynard JM, Peters TJ, Lim C, *et al*. The value of multiple free-flow studies in men with lower urinary tract symptoms. *Br J Urol* 1996; 7(6): 813-8.

25. Abrams P, Griffiths DJ. The assessment of prostatic obstruction from urodynamic measurements and from residual urine. *Br J Urol* 1979; 51: 129-34.

26. Jensen KME. Clinical evaluation of routine urodynamic investigation in prostates. *Neurourol Urodyn* 1989; 8: 545-78.

27. Rodrigues P, Lucon AM, Freire AC, Arap S. Urodynamic pressure flow studies can predict the clinical outcome after transurethral prostatic resection. *J Urol* 2001; 165: 499-502.

28. DeLancey G, Johnson S. Prostatism: how useful is routine imaging of the urinary tract?. *BMJ* 1988; 296: 965-967.

29. Choi J, Ikeguchi EF, Lee SW, *et al*. Is the higher prevalence of benign prostatic hyperplasia related to lower urinary tract symptoms in Korean men due to a high transition zone index? *Eur Urol* 2002; 42: 7-11.

30. Brawer MK, Abrahamsson PA, *et al*. Excluding prostate cancer in men presenting with lower urinary tract symptomatology (LUTS). In: *Benign Prostatic Hyperplasia*. Chatelain C, Denis L, Foo KT, *et al*, Eds. June 25-28, 2000. Health Publication Ltd, Plymouth, UK, 2001: 285-293.

31. Jacobsen SJ, Cynthia JG, Lieber MM. Natural history of benign prostatic hyperplasia. *Urology* 2001; 58, suppl 6A: 5-16.

32. Shoukry I, Susset JG, Elhilali MM, Dutartre D. Role of uroflometry in the assessment of lower urinary tract obstruction in adult males. *Br J Urol* 1975; 47(5): 559-66.

Chapter 12

Surgical therapy for symptomatic benign prostatic hyperplasia

Srinath Chandrasekera MS FRCS FEBU

Senior Research Fellow, Urology

Gordon Muir FRCS (Urol) FEBU

Consultant Urological Surgeon

KING'S COLLEGE HOSPITAL, LONDON, UK

Introduction

Although numerous treatment modalities are currently available for treating benign prostatic hyperplasia (BPH), surgery remains the final option for a significant proportion of patients. Approximately 30% of those with moderate to severe lower urinary tract symptoms due to symptomatic BPH will eventually need surgical intervention [1] **(II/B)**.

Transurethral resection of the prostate (TURP) has been regarded as the standard contemporary operation for BPH [1,2] **(IV/C)**. Strong indications for a prostatectomy include acute urinary retention, high-pressure chronic retention, recurrent urinary tract infections or bladder stones due to outflow obstruction and haematuria due to BPH [1,2]. However, with increasing safety demonstrated with surgery, these indications have been extended to symptoms such as poor flow, dribbling, hesitancy, incomplete emptying and other lower urinary tract symptoms caused by BPH [3,4] **(IV/C)**.

It has been shown that those with moderate symptoms of benign prostatic hyperplasia are more effectively treated with surgery than with watchful waiting [4] **(Ib/A)**. Approximately half the patients undergo prostatectomy in the UK due to urinary retention [5,6]. There have been major developments in alternate surgical therapies for symptomatic BPH in the last two decades. The aims of these techniques have been to reduce invasiveness and morbidity while retaining efficacy.

Methodology

This chapter reviews the different forms of surgical interventions available for symptomatic BPH, based on a Medline study.

Established surgical options for the treatment of symptomatic BPH include:

- Transurethral resection of the prostate (TURP).
- Transurethral incision of the prostate (TUIP).
- Transurethral vaporisation of the prostate (TUVP).
- Transurethral laser vaporisation.
- Transuretral holmium laser resection/enucleation.
- Open prostatectomy.

Open prostatectomy

Open prostatectomy was initially performed through a perineal route (this technique is obsolete now). The current retropubic prostatectomy was popularised by Millin although similar versions of this technique had been described earlier [7].

In the modern era, indications for open prostatectomy vary in different settings, the commonest being for large prostates (more than 80-100ml) [1]. The logic of this size trigger relates to the risk of significant irrigant absorption associated with longer resection times **(IIb/B)**. Another indication includes those who need open surgery for the treatment of large bladder stones untreatable by endoscopic means or large bladder diverticulae requiring surgical treatment, for whom a concurrent prostatectomy is planned. A combination of retropubic prostatectomy with extra-peritoneal hernia repair has been described, although this is not common practice. Open prostatectomy might be indicated due to the unavailability of transurethral instrumentation or indeed, expertise.

Transurethral resection of the prostate (TURP)

The first resectoscope that resembled the modern day transurethral instruments was invented in 1926 by Stern [7]. Although this technique initially suffered major morbidity, TURP was soon established as the standard worldwide procedure [3,7]. TURP is currently regarded by many as the gold standard operation for the relief of bladder outflow obstruction [1,2] **(IV/C)**. Although there is only one randomised controlled study comparing TURP with open prostatectomy to date [8], the results of TURP, in terms of symptom relief and improvement in urine flow, have been found to be broadly similar in single arm studies. In the National Prostatectomy Audit of the UK, (Emberton *et al*), 95% of the operations were either TURP or its variant, transurethral incision of the prostate [5].

The main limitation of TURP is its relative inability to resect larger glands over 80-100ml due to risks of transurethral resection syndrome. Although there are sporadic reports of TURP being performed as a catheter-free day-case procedure [9], this operation usually requires an in-dwelling catheter and hospital stay for a few days, with a transfusion risk of 4%-5% [4] **(Ib/A)**.

Transurethral electro-vaporisation (TUVP) and transurethral incision of the prostate (TUIP) can be considered variations of TURP, as identical or near identical instruments and energy sources are used [2]. TUIP and TUVP have therefore not been discussed separately in this chapter.

Alternate surgical therapies

The quest for interventions with equal efficacy, but less morbidity, has resulted in the development of new surgical technologies for treating symptomatic BPH since the 1980s [10]. In the new millennium, transurethral laser vaporisation and holmium laser prostatectomy are at the forefront of those techniques, challenging TURP for its gold standard status. Although the use of lasers for the treatment of BPH has been contemplated since the mid-80s, it was not until the '90s that this became common practice [1,2]. The initial laser procedures, despite early enthusiasm, fell into disrepute due to the high re-operation rates, which may be the cause of some of the scepticism regarding the newer generation lasers of the 21st Century. The techniques most frequently discussed at present seem to be the high power potassium titanyl phosphate (KTP) laser, and holmium laser enucleation (HoLEP) or resection (HoLRP).

The KTP laser system delivers light energy of a wavelength in the green visible spectrum. Light of this wavelength is absorbed preferentially by red tissue, such as haemoglobin or any blood-bearing tissue such as the prostate gland [11]. The KTP laser, having a minimum depth penetration, is poorly absorbed by water. KTP laser systems offer a virtually bloodless operating field with minimal surrounding coagulative necrosis [10,11]. As opposed to the low-powered Nd:YAG versions of the 1990s, which depended on coagulative necrosis and delayed sloughing of tissue which took four to six weeks, the current high-power delivery system results in immediate tissue vaporisation and therefore relief of obstruction [10,12]. Hospital stay and catheter time is minimal with this technique and it has been our own experience (unpublished data) that KTP laser prostatectomy can be performed safely as a day-case catheter-free procedure in selected patients. The main advantages of this technique are the relative bloodless field of operation and short hospital stay.

In a small series by Sandhu et al, the safety of KTP laser in dealing with large prostates has been demonstrated [13]. The complete absence of intra-operative irrigant absorption during this procedure is certainly facilitatory towards handling larger glands [14] **(IIb/B)**. Having operated on over 30 patients with prostates larger than 100mls, it is our experience that high-powered (80 watt) KTP laser vaporisation (PVP) is suitable for the treatment of very large glands.

Holmium laser prostatectomy using 60-80 watt systems can be carried out by employing varying techniques including holmium laser vaporisation, resection (HoLRP) or most recently, holmium laser enucleation (HoLEP) [1,15]. Unlike its low-powered precursors, which depended on tissue coagulation, the newer versions of holmium lasers have precise cutting abilities, resulting in the immediate creation of a TURP-like cavity with good levels of haemostasis [15,16]. The depth of energy penetration with holmium techniques is greater than the KTP system and is able to produce adequate haemostasis in vessels of 2mm [16-18] **(IIb/B)**.

The main advantage of holmium laser resection and enucleation seems to be excellent haemostasis, immediate relief of symptoms and its ability to deal with large prostate glands [15,19,20]. In a recent single-centre randomised study, Kuntz et al, demonstrated that transurethral holmium laser enucleation of the prostate (HoLEP) is a suitable and safe alternative to open prostatectomy [19] **(Ib/A)**.

Older generation lasers have the common limitations of the lack of immediate effect and the need for prolonged catheter drainage. These techniques are no longer recommended as suitable options for the treatment of BPH [1], unless under special circumstances when patients are unsuitable for TURP, open prostatectomy or high-powered laser therapy. These techniques will therefore not be discussed.

Safety and efficacy outcomes

When considering an optimal treatment method, safety and efficacy outcomes along with morbidity profiles, need to be considered. The newer techniques have been subjected to a much greater degree of scrutiny than TURP and open prostatectomy ever were. Most studies have focused on improvement in symptom scores and quality of life along with flow rates and residual urine volumes. Urodynamic aspects have been less well studied.

In the Veterans' Affairs Co-operative study, randomising patients with moderate to severe lower urinary tract symptoms (LUTS) between TURP and watchful waiting, TURP was more effective than watchful waiting for symptomatic relief [4] **(Ib/A)**.

In 1996, Emberton and Neal et al demonstrated the effect of TURP in significantly improving BPH-related symptoms and bother [21] **(III/B)**. The follow-up period was short in the study and the pre-operative symptoms were recalled three months following surgery. Only 75% of those with mild to moderate symptoms were satisfied following surgery, as opposed to 90% of those with strong indications. TUIP and TUVP have had similar results **(III/B)**.

The mean improvement of LUTS following TURP in 29 randomised studies with a TURP arm as treatment was found to be 71% (range 66%-76%) [1,22] **(Ia/A)**. The mean increase of flow rate (Qmax) following TURP was 115% (range 80%-150%) [22]. The improvement in maximum flow rates has been best with open prostatectomy (175%), which improves flow by 8.2-22.6ml/sec [23-25] **(IIb/B)**.

Results of laser vaporisation of the prostate are mostly based on the 60 watt hybrid technique. Carter, in a randomised trial, has demonstrated that the 60 watt KTP laser vaporisation is as effective as TURP in improving symptoms as well as flow rates at one year [26] **(Ib/A)**. In our own non-randomised series of 50 patients undergoing 80 watt PVP, the mean improvement of symptoms in terms of IPSS score was 21 to 6.8 with a reduction in the mean quality of life score from 4.6 to 1.2.

Most of the information regarding holmium laser prostatectomy is derived from the work of Gilling et al.

In a systemic review of holmium laser prostatectomy for benign prostatic hyperplasia, Tooher *et al* conclude that there was no overall difference in the maximum flow rates achieved at six months between holmium laser prostatectomy and TURP [15] **(Ia/A)**. These findings were based on pooled data from three randomised studies [27-29]. However, when the results of holmium laser resection were separated from holmium laser enucleation of the prostate, a significant difference in favour of holmium laser resection compared to TURP has been demonstrated **(Ib/A)**. In the same review, there were no differences in symptom relief demonstrable between holmium prostatectomy and TURP [15,30]. Similar conclusions have been derived by the single arm meta-analyses conducted by the American Urology Association (AUA) [2]. In this study, the mean reduction of symptoms is 15 points for holmium prostatectomy, TURP and laser vaporisation. Peak flow rates at 16 months were not significantly different between TURP, holmium prostatectomy, laser vaporisation and open prostatectomy, although open prostatectomy performed best with a maximum flow rate increase of 14ml/sec **(III/B)**.

The mortality data comparing different techniques are sparse. This is probably due to the rarity of the event, particularly with the newer techniques. The mortality following TURP for elective indications was 0.2%, significantly differing for those who undergo surgery following retention (0.8%) ($p<0.02$) [6] **(III/B)**.

The mean hospital stay following TURP has been noted to be four days [4]. Kuntz, in a randomised study of TURP versus holmium enucleation of the prostate, demonstrated that the hospital stay was significantly reduced with holmium enucleation of the prostate (two versus three days in favour of HoLEP) [15] **(Ib/A)**.

The mean duration of catheterisation was shorter with holmium resection as opposed to TURP, although this translated to only 0.8 days for holmium laser resection and 1.2 days shorter for holmium laser enucleation [15] **(Ib/A)**. The mean hospital stay following PVP was 1.5 days [31]. In our institution we carry out most PVPs as a day-case procedure where postoperative catheters are used only on an individualised basis. In summary, symptomatic improvement, as well as improvements in flow rates,

is largely similar between TURP, open prostatectomy, photo-selective vaporisation and holmium prostatectomy. Hospital stay seems to be significantly lower with newer interventional techniques with reduced catheter times. There is insufficient data on mortality, probably due to the rarity of the event.

Adverse events

The following adverse events were cited in the literature.

- TURP syndrome.
- Blood transfusion.
- Haematuria.
- Irritative lower urinary tract symptoms.
- Urinary tract infections.
- Re-operation.
- Urethral/bladder neck stricture.
- Urinary incontinence.
- Retrograde ejaculation/sexual dysfunction.

Intra-operative complications

The meta-analysis carried out by the AUA reveals that overall intra-operative complication rates are less than 3% for those treated with TURP, transurethral electro-vaporisation and laser vaporisation [2] **(III/B)**. Those undergoing TURP for acute retention were found to have an increased risk of peri-operative complications, although large prostate size (resected weight more than 40g) and associated comorbidity (ASA grade more than 2) were notable confounding variables [5,6] **(III/B)**. When these factors were taken into account, the association of those with acute retention was less significant ($p<0.04$). More importantly, increased operative time (more than one hour), blood loss and difficulty during surgery were notable associations with major postoperative morbidity [5] **(III/B)**. Similar information on newer techniques is lacking. In a contemporary series on 32 transvesical prostatectomies, Tubaro *et al* found no mortality **(III/B)**, although intra-operative events are not clearly documented [23].

Haematuria and transfusion

Haematuria seems to be an ill-defined complication; therefore, conclusive information is difficult to gather. The Veterans' Affairs Co-operative study reports a transfusion rate of 4%-5% following TURP [4] **(Ib/A)**. The frequency of transfusions for TUIP, electro-vaporisation and laser prostatectomy have been found to be significantly lower than TURP in the AUA meta-analysis [2].

In a randomised controlled trial comparing transurethral holmium laser enucleation (HoLEP) with open prostatectomy in 120 patients with prostates larger than 100g, no patient in the holmium laser arm required transfusion, as opposed to eight in the open prostatectomy group [19]. However, in this study the transfusion trigger is not defined. Similarly, Carter, in a prospective trial comparing hybrid laser versus TURP on 204 patients, noted a 0% transfusion requirement for laser vaporisation as opposed to 5% in the TURP arm [26] **(Ib/A)**. Transfusion is not usually required for other interventional techniques [1,2] **(IV/C)**.

In summary, the risk of blood transfusion is significantly higher in those who undergo open prostatectomy or TURP.

Lower Urinary Tract Symptoms (LUTS)

Short to medium-term irritative lower urinary tract symptoms following older laser techniques have been one of its major drawbacks [1,2]. These include dysuria, urinary frequency, urgency and urge incontinence. However, the newer techniques seem to have overcome this shortcoming to a great extent due to their ability to produce immediate tissue ablation rather than coagulative necrosis with delayed tissue sloughing seen with older low-powered methods. Although irritative lower urinary tract symptoms were significantly higher in those who underwent 60 watt KTP laser vaporisation, at six weeks (p<0.01), these changes were not significant at a follow-up interval of one year [26] **(Ib/A)**. Cairn and Gilling in a randomised trial comparing HoLEP and TURP in 61 patients, did not find significant differences in LUTS at one year [20] **(Ib/A)**. Similar conclusions have been derived by the AUA meta-analysis based on randomised controlled studies [2]. Of note is that the incidence of these events documented in a single series, have a wide variation.

Urinary tract infections

The category of urinary tract infections (UTI) includes a variety of problems, such as wound infection, urethroprostatitis, epididymitis and orchitis.

Tubaro *et al* documents urinary tract infections in 12.5% and wound infection in 3.1% of the 32 patients undergoing suprapubic transvesical prostatectomy [23] **(III/B)**. Urinary tract infections following laser vaporisation have been notably higher. Carter *et al* found that the incidence of urinary tract infections was almost twice as common with laser vaporisation than with a TURP [26] **(Ib/A)**. The incidence of urinary tract infection following holmium prostatectomy is less clearly documented. However, the AUA meta-analysis based on randomised controlled studies, revealed no statistically significant differences in the rates of UTI in patients treated with transurethral laser coagulation, TURP and electro-vaporisation [2] **(Ib/A)**.

Urinary incontinence

Urinary incontinence represents a group of adverse events, which may be total or partial incontinence, stress incontinence or urge incontinence. The frequency of urinary incontinence following TURP has been calculated to be 3% [2]. In the national prostatectomy audit, 33% of those who were continent pre-operatively were incontinent three months following TURP. Only 6% of those reported this to be problematic requiring the wearing of pads. These figures improved to 1% at six months [21] **(III/B)**. In Tubaro's series, 9.4% of those who underwent transvesical prostatectomy were noted to have temporary stress incontinence, which resolved at three months [23] **(III/B)**. There have been no significant differences in urinary incontinence between holmium laser enucleation and TURP [15] **(Ib/A)**. There are insufficient data comparing laser vaporisation and TURP to make any statement in this area.

The figures from the AUA also did not find any statistical significant differences in urinary incontinence between TURP, holmium laser resection or open prostatectomy [2].

Bladder neck/urethral stricture

The rate of bladder neck stricture has been suggested to be higher with TURP and open prostatectomy compared to laser techniques [1]. However, numerous other analyses do not reveal statistically significant differences between any of these techniques [2,15]. The risk of bladder neck contracture has been documented to be 1.8% after open prostatectomy, 4% after TURP and 0.4% after TUIP [1] (III/B). Reports on bladder neck contracture following laser techniques are inconsistent, although there has not been any notable difference between these and TURP.

Sexual dysfunction

Sexual dysfunction following prostatectomy may occur in the form of erectile dysfunction (ED) or ejaculatory dysfunction. In the Veterans' Affairs Co-operative study, the occurrence of erectile dysfunction was found to be lower in the TURP group than with watchful waiting [4] (Ib/A). The estimated frequency of ED has been calculated to be 10% following TURP. This has been noted to be higher (31%) by Emberton, who also reported that approximately two-thirds of men experienced retrograde ejaculation following TURP [21] (III/B). The reporting of sexual dysfunction in studies comparing KTP vaporisation and holmium prostatectomy has been rather inconsistent. The incidence of retrograde ejaculation has been found to be almost similar with holmium enucleation and open prostatectomy. Reports on erectile dysfunction are difficult to evaluate in these series, as they seem to be based mostly on subjective evaluation.

Meta-analyses of RCTs have found no statistical significant differences in the rates of erectile dysfunction between TURP and laser vaporisation. The AUA analysis revealed that the lowest rate of ejaculatory dysfunction was with transurethral laser coagulation and TUIP (17%-18%) with no differences demonstrated between laser vaporisation and TURP [2].

Catheter time and re-catheterisation

Open prostatectomy and conventional transurethral resection of the prostate require an in-dwelling catheter, often with continuous bladder irrigation. In a contemporary series by Tubaro, the approximate catheter time was five days following open transvesical prostatectomy [23]. A notable advantage of newer techniques has been the shorter catheter time. Malek, in a prospective series of KTP laser vaporisation, documented a mean catheter time of 20 hours [32] (IIb/B).

In a systematic review of holmium laser prostatectomy for BPH, Tooher notes significant differences in the catheter protocols in different studies, which makes comparison rather inaccurate. However, based on analysis of studies suitable for comparison, the mean catheterisation time was 0.8 days shorter for holmium laser resection than with TURP [15] (Ia/A).

Evidence on re-catheterisation rates is conflicting. In the national prostatectomy audit, 2.3% of those who underwent TURP for lower urinary tract symptoms, required re-catheterisation, as opposed to 9.2% of those with acute retention. Of these patients, 0.1% and 0.9% required a permanent catheter respectively [5] (III/B). In a separate non-randomised series by Malek, none of the patients undergoing high-powered KTP laser vaporisation required re-catheterisation [31]. However, in a randomised study comparing the low-powered 60 watt KTP versus TURP, a significantly higher proportion of those who underwent KTP laser vaporisation (32%) required re-catheterisation as opposed to 5% following TURP (Ib/A).

Hoffman and Richard et al in a systematic review, noted a significant difference in urinary retention rates between laser techniques and TURP in favour of the latter [20] (Ia/A). Similar conclusions have been arrived at following the data analysis of the American Urology Association [2].

In summary, interpretation of data on catheter times and urinary retention is difficult, as hardly any study described catheterisation protocols. However, in the majority of studies, catheter time following surgery is reduced following laser techniques, although the re-catheterisation rates are significantly higher when compared with TURP **(Ib/A)**.

Conclusions

Surgery for symptomatic benign prostatic hyperplasia is one of the commonest operations performed in the ageing male. Open prostatectomy was the dominant operation in the earlier half of the 20th Century. With the development of optics, TURP became the preferred treatment and is regarded by most (without what is now regarded as "hard" evidence) as the benchmark surgical therapy for symptomatic BPH. A survey of the literature shows that TURP was established mostly due to individual experiences, as only one randomised study comparing TURP to open prostatectomy exists. However, the perceived advantages of a minimal access and thus a less morbid technique seem overwhelming. Nevertheless, the reality of the morbidity associated with TURP has led to the search for procedures that are still less invasive and hence less morbid, whilst retaining the outcomes seen with open prostatectomy or TURP. This being the era of evidence-based medical practice, the newer techniques have necessarily been subjected to greater scrutiny. Many of these studies have utilised TURP in their control arms, although the endpoints and time frames have varied widely in many of these studies.

Although some of the earlier heat-based and laser interventions have now fallen out of favour due to perceived inferior results, the newer generation high-powered versions seem to show equal, if not better outcomes, compared to TURP. In this respect, the newer techniques, such as high-powered KTP laser vaporisation and holmium laser prostatectomy give better outcomes in terms of hospital stay, catheter time and transfusion rates. Symptom relief and improvements in flow are comparable to TURP. In selected patients, the KTP laser may offer further benefits, with the potential of being a totally catheter-free procedure carried out as a true day-case, further minimising the impact of surgical treatment on the quality of life of the patient.

One of the dominant drawbacks of a conventional TURP was its relative inability to handle larger prostate glands. This seems to have been overcome by the newer lasers, which may potentially make open prostatectomy obsolete.

Whilst there are excellent long-term randomised data on HoLEP, all from a limited number of centres, demonstrating the equivalence and indeed, superiority of this technique over TURP, longer-term results for the new generation high-powered KTP techniques are awaited. Whilst one could argue that most studies on TURP only have a follow-up of one year at best, longer follow-up times with newer techniques would certainly be more convincing.

Although randomised controlled studies may produce the best evidence, there are serious concerns about the logistics and ethics of such studies in new surgical techniques [33,34]. The fact that surgical trials can never be double blind introduces the significant possibility of operator bias in the analysis of any new technique. Similar problems may arise when comparing TURP with the newer laser techniques, where in certain instances novel surrogate endpoints, as well as general acceptance of a new technique, may need to be considered for more appropriate measures of success in this new millennium of medical care.

Chapter 12

Recommendations	Evidence level

♦ "Absolute" indications for surgery for BPH are: **III/B**
  - Refractory urinary retention.
  - High pressure chronic retention.
  - Complications such as recurrent haematuria, bladder stones, UTI and bladder diverteculae caused by outflow obstruction due to BPH.

♦ "Relative" indications extend to those with bothersome LUTS, as those with mild to moderate symptoms are more effectively treated with TURP than watchful waiting. **Ib/A**

♦ TURP is considered the standard surgical therapy for BPH. **III/B**

♦ Holmium laser enucleation/resection is a suitable alternative to open prostatectomy in the treatment of adenomas >100ml. **Ib/A**

♦ In expert hands, advantages of high-powered holmium laser techniques are reduced hospital stay, blood transfusions and catheter time while achieving comparable symptom relief and flow rates. Although high-power KTP laser vaporisation also shows great promise in all these domains, long-term data are not available for definitive conclusions. **Ib/A**

References

1. Rosette J, Madersbacher S, Alivizatos G, Rioja Sanz C, Emberton M, Nordling J. Guidelines on Benign Prostatic Hyperplasia. http://www.uroweb.org/index.php?structure_id=140. 2004.

2. Management of BPH. American Urological Association Education and Research, Inc. 2003. http://healthcommunities.com/mdonly/pdf/chapt_3_appendix.pdf.

3. Neal DE. The National Prostatectomy Audit. Br J Urol 1997; 79 Suppl 2: 69-75.

4. Wasson JH, Reda DJ, Bruskewitz RC, Elinson J, Keller AM, Henderson WG. A comparison of transurethral surgery with watchful waiting for moderate symptoms of benign prostatic hyperplasia. The Veterans Affairs Cooperative Study Group on Transurethral Resection of the Prostate. N Engl J Med 1995; 332(2): 75-79.

5. Pickard R, Emberton M, Neal DE. The management of men with acute urinary retention. National Prostatectomy Audit Steering Group. Br J Urol 1998; 81(5): 712-720.

6. Emberton M, Neal DE, Black N, Harrison M, Fordham M, McBrien MP, et al. The National Prostatectomy Audit: the clinical management of patients during hospital admission. Br J Urol 1995; 75(3): 301-316.

7. Murphy LJT. The Prostate. In: The History of Urology. Murphy LJT, Ed. Charles C Thomas, Springfield, Illinois, USA, 1972: 378-452.

8. Meyhoff HH, Nordling J, Hald T. Clinical evaluation of transurethral versus transvesical prostatectomy. A randomized study. Scand J Urol Nephrol 1984; 18(3): 201-209.

9. Chander J, Vanitha V, Lal P, Ramteke VK. Transurethral resection of the prostate as catheter-free day-care surgery. BJU Int 2003; 92(4): 422-425.

10. Anson K. Could the latest generation potassium titanyl phosphate lasers be the ones to make transurethral resection of the prostate an operation of historical interest only? Curr Opin Urol 2004; 14(1): 27-29.

11. Barber NJ, Muir GH. High-power KTP laser prostatectomy: the new challenge to transurethral resection of the prostate. Curr Opin Urol 2004; 14(1): 21-25.

12. van Melick HH, van Venrooij GE, Eckhardt MD, Boon TA. A randomized controlled trial comparing transurethral resection of the prostate, contact laser prostatectomy and electrovaporization in men with benign prostatic hyperplasia: urodynamic effects. J Urol 2002; 168(3): 1058-1062.

13. Sandhu J, Vanderbrink B, Egan C, Kaplan S, Te A. High-power KTP photoselective laser vaporisation prostatectomy for the treatment of benign prostatic hyperplasia in men with large prostates. J Urol 2003; 169(4): 393.

14. Barber NJ, Zhu G, Donohue J, Thompson PM, Walsh K, Muir GH. The evaluation of irrigant absorption during high power KTP laser vaporization of the prostate by the use of expired breath ethanol. Br J Urol 2004; 93(4): 106.

15. Tooher R, Sutherland P, Costello A, Gilling P, Rees G, Maddern G. A systematic review of holmium laser prostatectomy for benign prostatic hyperplasia. J Urol 2004; 171(5): 1773-1781.

16. Erhard MJ, Bagley DH. Urologic applications of the holmium laser: preliminary experience. J Endourol 1995; 9(5): 383-386.

17. Le DA, Gilling PJ. Holmium laser resection of the prostate. *Eur Urol* 1999; 35(2): 155-160.

18. Wollin TA, Denstedt JD. The holmium laser in urology. *J Clin Laser Med Surg* 1998; 16(1): 13-20.

19. Kuntz RM, Lehrich K. Transurethral holmium laser enucleation versus transvesical open enucleation for prostate adenoma greater than 100 gm: a randomized prospective trial of 120 patients. *J Urol* 2002; 168(4 Pt1): 1465-1469.

20. Hoffman RM, MacDonald R, Slaton JW, Wilt TJ. Laser prostatectomy versus transurethral resection for treating benign prostatic obstruction: a systematic review. *J Urol* 2003; 169(1): 210-215.

21. Emberton M, Neal DE, Black N, Fordham M, Harrison M, McBrien MP, *et al*. The effect of prostatectomy on symptom severity and quality of life. *Br J Urol* 1996; 77(2): 233-247.

22. Madersbacher S, Marberger M. Is transurethral resection of the prostate still justified? *BJU Int* 1999; 83(3): 227-237.

23. Tubaro A, Carter S, Hind A, Vicentini C, Miano L. A prospective study of the safety and efficacy of suprapubic transvesical prostatectomy in patients with benign prostatic hyperplasia. *J Urol* 2001; 166(1): 172-176.

24. Mearini E, Marzi M, Mearini L, Zucchi A, Porena M. Open prostatectomy in benign prostatic hyperplasia: 10-year experience in Italy. *Eur Urol* 1998; 34(6): 480-485.

25. Serretta V, Morgia G, Fondacaro L, Curto G, Lo BA, Pirritano D, *et al*. Open prostatectomy for benign prostatic enlargement in southern Europe in the late 1990s: a contemporary series of 1800 interventions. *Urology* 2002; 60(4): 623-627.

26. Carter A, Sells H, Speakman M, Ewings P, MacDonagh R, O'Boyle P. A prospective randomized controlled trial of hybrid laser treatment or transurethral resection of the prostate, with a 1-year follow-up. *BJU Int* 1999; 83(3): 254-259.

27. Gilling P, Kennett K, Fraundorfer MR. Holmium laser enucleation of the prostate (HoLEP) is superior to TURP for the relief of bladder outflow obstruction (BOO). *J Endourol* 2001.

28. Hammad FT, Mark SD, Davidson PJ, Gowland SP, Gordon B, English SF. Holmium: YAG laser resection versus transurethral resection of the prostate: a randomized prospective trial with 1-year follow-up. *ANZ J Surg* 2002; 72(A): 138.

29. Tan AH, Gilling PJ. Holmium laser prostatectomy. *BJU Int* 2003; 92(6): 527-530.

30. Gilling PJ, Mackey M, Cresswell M, Kennett K, Kabalin JN, Fraundorfer MR. Holmium laser versus transurethral resection of the prostate: a randomized prospective trial with 1-year follow-up. *J Urol* 1999; 162(5): 1640-1644.

31. Larner T, Nawrocki J. Photoselective vaporization of the prostate for BPH. Outcome at 3 months in our first 50 unselected patients. *BJU Int* 2004; 93(4):110.

32. Malek RS, Kuntzman RS, Barrett DM. High power potassium-titanyl-phosphate laser vaporization prostatectomy. *J Urol* 2000; 163(6): 1730-1733.

33. Jenkins BJ, Sharma P, Badenoch DF, Fowler CG, Blandy JP. Ethics, logistics and a trial of transurethral versus open prostatectomy. *Br J Urol* 1992; 69(4): 372-374.

34. Roos NP, Wennberg JE, Malenka DJ, Fisher ES, McPherson K, Andersen TF, *et al*. Mortality and reoperation after open and transurethral resection of the prostate for benign prostatic hyperplasia. *N Engl J Med* 1989; 320(17): 1120-1124.

Chapter 12

Surgical therapy for symptomatic
benign prostatic hyperplasia

Chapter 13

Screening for prostate cancer

Oliver Wiseman MA FRCS

Specialist Registrar, Urology

EDITH CAVELL HOSPITAL, PETERBOROUGH, UK

Introduction

Screening can be defined as the performance of tests, in a population of asymptomatic individuals, to detect unrecognised disease with the intention of thereafter modifying the natural history of the disease through treatment to the benefit of the individual concerned. Screening programmes which have been implemented are based upon the general principles of screening which were formulated in 1968 by Wilson and Jungner for the World Health Organisation (Table 1) [1]. It has been pointed out, however, that these criteria do not specify the need for evidence from randomised trials, give no guide whether a screening programme should be implemented if certain criteria are only partly met, and indicate that the decision to screen should be based on a series of binary options when screening is in fact a programme of risk reduction where all criteria should interact [2].

There are three ways of screening for disease. The first is by mass screening, which is a comprehensive screening program in a population which may be defined in terms of, for example, sex and/or age. The second is selective screening, which targets only high risk populations. Finally, screening may be opportunistic, which involves testing individual patients using screening instruments. It is opportunistic screening that is currently undertaken by many urologists for prostate cancer, as national screening programmes do not currently exist. This chapter will concentrate only on the evidence for introducing a mass screening programme for the detection of prostate cancer, and in examining this evidence it will be structured according to the general principles of screening as laid out by Wilson and Jungner [1].

Does prostate cancer pose an important health problem?

Prostate cancer is an important health problem, with an annual incidence of over 21,000 in the UK, and a mortality of almost 9,500 [3]. In the USA, prostate cancer is the second leading cause of cancer death to lung cancer, with an estimated 220,000 new cases diagnosed and over 28,000 deaths in 2003 [4] **(IV/C)**.

Table 1. Principles of screening for disease [1].

- The condition sought should be an important health problem
- The natural history of the condition, including development from latent to declared disease, should be well understood
- There should be a recognisable latent or early stage
- There should be an accepted treatment for patients with recognised disease
- There should be a suitable test or examination to detect the disease
- The test should be acceptable to the population
- Facilities for diagnosis and treatment should be available
- There should be an agreed policy on whom to treat as patients
- Screening should be repeated at intervals determined by the natural history of the disease
- The cost, including diagnosis and treatment of patients diagnosed, should be economically balanced in relation to possible expenditure on medical care as a whole

Is the natural history of the disease well understood?

The natural history of prostate cancer is uncertain, as we know that men are much more likely to die with prostate cancer, rather than from it. The lifetime risk of having microscopic prostate cancer for a man of 50 years is 42%, whereas the risk of dying from it is only 3% [5]. Thus, the cancer is latent in the vast majority of individuals, and the difficulty comes in identifying which cancers are clinically significant. The size of the tumour and Gleason grade have been shown to be important prognostic indicators.

Studies where incidental tumours were discovered at the time of surgery for benign prostatic hyperplasia, have shown that the risk of progression in patients where less than 5% of the surgical specimen contains cancer was 5% at five years, 15%-20% at ten years, and approximately 30% at 15 years. Less than 10% of such patients will die from their cancer. This is in contrast to patients where tumour volume was greater than 5% of the specimen where the risk of mortality is much higher [6].

A further prognostic indicator comes from the Gleason grade. In Albertsen's risk analysis of men with prostate cancer aged 55-74, who were treated conservatively, the chance of dying from the disease within 15 years was 4%-7% for those with Gleason 2-4 tumours, 18%-30% for those with Gleason 6 tumours, and 60%-87% for those with Gleason scores 8-10 [7].

Is there a suitable test?

There are difficulties in defining the characteristics of a suitable test in screening for prostate cancer, and any figures which are given define their accuracy based upon findings at needle biopsy, an invasive diagnostic test which may miss cancers that are present, find cancers which are unrelated to abnormal screening results, and not necessarily identify those patients who have clinically significant disease. Screening can be undertaken using digital rectal examination (DRE), serum prostate specific antigen (PSA) testing, transrectal ultrasound (TRUS) and biopsy of the prostate, or combinations of all three.

Digital Rectal Exam (DRE)

DRE was the test used for the detection of prostate cancer prior to the 1990s, but is limited by the fact that only the posterior and lateral parts of the gland can be palpated. Twenty to thirty-five percent of tumours may occur in portions of the gland not accessible on DRE [8, 9]. Furthermore, it has limited reproducibility [10].

The positive predictive value of DRE alone has been shown to be between 21% and 28% [11-13] which is low. This leads to a high biopsy rate, increasing anxiety and morbidity, as well as high cost for the screened population. One of these studies showed that cancer was detected in 1.1% of the screened population [12], and in another randomised study, this percentage was 2.4% [14]. As we will see, these levels are lower than those found with PSA testing and this, together with its low positive predictive value, must indicate that DRE has little value as a mass screening method.

Prostate Specific Antigen (PSA)

A more promising screening test is measurement of serum PSA. PSA is a serine protease that is a tissue-specific marker, but not cancer-specific, and is raised in conditions such as urinary tract infection, benign prostatic hyperplasia, and after urinary tract instrumentation as well as in prostate cancer.

In the Physician's health study, using a PSA cut-off point of 4.0 or higher, the sensitivity for detecting cancer appearing within two years after screening was 73% [15]. Other studies have found similar results [16, 17]. The positive predictive value is 10% in those with a PSA of <4.0ng/ml, and approximately 25% and 50%-67% in those with a PSA of 4-10 and >10ng/ml respectively [18, 19]. Specificity of PSA testing at a cut-off of 4.0ng/ml may be as high as 91% [15], while others suggest it may be between 60%-70% [20].

As well as detecting more tumours than DRE, PSA testing also detects these tumours earlier. Prior to the introduction of PSA screening, up to 35% of patients with what was thought to be clinically localised prostate cancer had involved lymph nodes [21], and two thirds had pathologically advanced disease [22]. Since the advent of PSA testing, lymph node involvement may be as low as 5% [23], and annual testing has been shown to reduce the number of patients with clinically advanced disease [24]. In one study where the characteristics of screen detected cancers using DRE, PSA and TRUS were compared to cases discovered prior to screening, significant stage reduction of prostate cancer was shown to be afforded by screening, with 77% of cancers being organ-confined, and under 1% of patients having lymph node and metastatic involvement each [25]. Other studies have shown PSA screen detected cancers may be clinically localised in 85% of cases [26].

Combining the findings of DRE and PSA increases the positive predictive value, as shown in Table 2. With a PSA less than 4ng/ml, the chance of finding cancer on biopsy varies from 4%-9% if the DRE is negative; to up to 21% if it is positive [27, 28]. However, for a PSA greater than 4ng/ml, the chance is up to 32% if DRE is negative [11], and as high as 72% if DRE findings are positive [28], though in one of the largest studies it was lower at 55% [29].

Traditionally, 4ng/ml has been used as the upper limit of normal for PSA, but a number of cancers will be missed if this level is used. In one community-based study, 22% of men older than 50 years with PSAs between 2.6 and 4.0ng/ml had prostate cancer [30]. In the ERSPC trial, it is estimated that 63.5% of detectable cancers may not have been detected by

Chapter 13

Table 2. Chance of finding cancer on biopsy according to DRE findings and serum PSA.

Study	No of patients	PSA <4ng/ml DRE -ve	PSA <4ng/ml DRE +ve	PSA >4ng/ml DRE -ve	PSA >4ng/ml DRE +ve
Cooner et al, 1990 [27]	1807	9	17	25	62
Hammerer et al, 1994 [28]	651	4	21	12	72
Catalona et al, 1994 [11]	6630	-	10	32	49
Schroder et al, 1998 [29]	10523	-	13	-	55

using a PSA cut-off of 4.0ng/ml, and 87% of the screened population had PSA levels under 4.0ng/ml [17]. Furthermore, of those tumours detected at low PSAs, approximately half had aggressive characteristics [17]. Because of this, it has been suggested that the level for the cut-off be reduced from 4.0 to either 3.0 or even 2.6 [17, 31], thus resulting in more biopsies and more cancers detected [31].

In an attempt to improve the sensitivity of PSA screening and thus increase the number of cancers detected, and improve the specificity to decrease the number of unnecessary biopsies, a number of modifications of PSA testing have been introduced.

PSA velocity

Measurement of the rate of change of PSA with time, PSA velocity, was introduced in 1992 to try and improve the specificity of PSA testing [32]. Significant velocity differences between men with cancer and those with benign disease could be detected up to nine years before prostate cancer diagnosis, and it was concluded that an annual rise of PSA level of >0.75ng/ml warranted a prostate biopsy [32]. Another study followed 1,249 men screened by PSA and concluded that patients with a 20% annual increase in their PSA level should undergo further evaluation [33]. While measurement of PSA velocity does have its limitations, it is useful to assess the risk of prostate cancer in an individual whose PSA is between 4-10ng/ml, if there are three serial PSA measurements spanning at least a two-year time frame.

PSA density

The calculation of PSA density is an attempt to correct PSA values for volume of the gland, with the knowledge that prostate cancer releases more PSA per unit volume into the circulation than does BPH. This should allow better differentiation between prostate cancer and BPH in those with intermediate PSA levels. It is defined as the total serum PSA level divided by the transrectal ultrasound determined prostate volume. While early evidence suggested that this measure may help discriminate between patients with cancer and those with benign disease [34], and subsequent studies

Table 3. Recommended age-specific PSA reference ranges.

Age range	PSA reference range
40–49	0.0–2.5
50–59	0.0–3.5
60–69	0.0–4.5
70–79	0.0–6.5

reported that a PSA density enhanced the detection of cancer using a PSA density cut-off of 0.15 [35], others have found that 50% of prostate cancers would be missed using such a cut-off [36]. As the major determinant of serum PSA in men without prostate cancer is the transition zone epithelium, it has been suggested that adjusting PSA for transition zone volume (PSA-TZ) may help distinguish between BPH and prostate cancer [37], but while it has been shown that a cut-off value for the PSA-TZ of 0.35 provides a high positive predictive value for prostate cancer detection [38], lack of reproducibility makes this an investigational tool only at the present time.

Age-adjusted PSA

It is known that men without prostate cancer will have higher PSA values as they grow older, due to the growth of BPH tissue. In order to try and improve prostate cancer detection sensitivity in younger men and specificity in older men, Oesterling proposed age-related PSA reference ranges [39], as shown in Table 3. One large screening study of over 21,000 men aged 45-75 years found an 8% increase in the number of positive biopsies and organ-confined cancers in men under 60 using age-specific PSA ranges, and also a 21% decrease in biopsies of men over 60 years, while missing only 4% of organ-confined tumours [40]. However, the increased negative biopsy rate in younger patients, coupled with the possibility of missing cancers in the older age group has prevented uniform acceptance of this approach.

Complexed PSA and percent free PSA

Serum PSA exists in both free form and complexed to a number of protease inhibitors, especially α-1 antichymotrypsin. Assays for total PSA measure both free and complexed forms, but free PSA can be measured separately and the probability of having prostate cancer increases as the percentage of free PSA decreases [41, 42]. While the percent free PSA can increase the sensitivity of cancer detection for values under 4.0ng/ml, it is most often used to increase the specificity for patients whose total PSA lies between 4.0-10.0ng/ml. Most authors suggest a cut-off point of between 20 and 25 for percent-free PSA [43], and show that this might eliminate between 19%-64% of negative biopsies. Catalona investigated the sensitivities and specificities at various cut-off points, and showed that at a cut-off of 25% there was a 95% specificity and biopsies would have been avoided in 20% of patients [44]. Overall, the usefulness of the test is still to be fully determined, and one of the problems is that although it may provide additional information which represents a decrease in a man's probability of having prostate cancer, it is uncertain whether the reduction is low enough to mean that men and their physicians would be willing to avoid a biopsy.

In summary, PSA testing has a high sensitivity and specificity for the detection of prostate cancer **(IIb/B)**, and is more sensitive than DRE, but should be used in combination with it to increase the positive predictive value. Use of PSA testing allows the identification of more organ-confined tumours **(III/B)**, but modifications to its use to try and improve specificity and sensitivity remain unproven and at present there is no consensus on their use.

Transrectal Ultrasound (TRUS)

Transrectal ultrasound has a low sensitivity and specificity with regard to the values necessary for screening [45]. Its positive predictive value may be as low as 15.2% however [11], and is relatively expensive, as well as being less acceptable to patients compared to a blood test or DRE. It is thus only used in the diagnostic work up of a patient with an abnormal DRE or PSA, in conjunction with biopsies.

Effectiveness of current treatments for prostate cancer

Mass screening of asymptomatic members of the general public for prostate cancer is only worthwhile if we know that treatment will be of benefit. Indeed, Wilson and Jungner stated that "of all the criteria that a screening test should fulfil, the ability to treat the condition adequately, when discovered, is perhaps the most important" [1]. Thus, it is important to consider the effectiveness of the treatment options for early prostate cancer which consist of watchful waiting, or active surveillance, radiotherapy, interstitial brachytherapy and radical prostatectomy.

Despite the large numbers of men with early prostate cancer, we have very little good evidence on which to base our treatment decisions [2, 46]. Many studies comparing treatments are small, observational, or poorly conducted. Thus, recently published data from a randomised control trial by Holmberg *et al* comparing radical prostatectomy to watchful waiting is very important [47]. Over a ten-year period they randomly assigned 695 men with early, well or moderately differentiated prostate cancer to watchful waiting or radical prostatectomy, and had a median follow-up of over six years. They showed that radical prostatectomy reduced disease-specific mortality at eight years, rates of local progression and distant metastases, but did not show any difference in overall survival **(Ib/A)**. A difference in overall mortality might be expected to be seen as the study progresses, given the difference in disease-specific mortality, local progression and development of distant metastases seen at eight years. However, the population studied was different from those who would normally be identified by screening, as 76% of them had palpable tumours, so while this evidence is the best we currently have, it cannot be applied directly as evidence for or against screening.

While there are no other randomised controlled trials, we have other data to help inform us on the relative effectiveness of the treatment options. One observational study showed that for men with well differentiated cancer, ten-year disease-specific survival did not differ between those who underwent radical prostatectomy, or those who had radiation treatment or watchful waiting. However, disease-specific survival was much higher for men with poorly differentiated cancer, and slightly higher for men with moderately differentiated tumours [48] compared to both radiotherapy and watchful waiting **(III/B)**.

A large cohort study examined the biochemical relapse-free survival of 1865 patients treated between 1990 and 1998 with either radical radiotherapy or radical prostatectomy [49]. When these patients' tumours were segregated into two risk groups according to stage, Gleason score and PSA levels, no significant difference was found between those treated with surgery or radical radiotherapy for either favourable or unfavourable tumours. However, for patients with unfavourable tumours, radical radiotherapy at a dose of greater than 72Gy was better than both radical surgery and radical radiotherapy at a dose of less than 72Gy, and radical surgery was better than radical radiotherapy at a dose of less than 72Gy. The benefit of higher doses of radical radiotherapy in patients with a PSA >10ng/ml have been confirmed in a well conducted randomised study which also used biochemical failure as an endpoint [50]. However, biochemical failure has been shown not be an independent predictor of mortality at ten years after either radical prostatectomy or radical radiotherapy [51, 52] and thus while it may give us some idea of comparative treatment efficacies, it is possibly not evidence directly applicable to the screening debate.

There is no well conducted randomised controlled trial comparing external beam radiotherapy to other treatments for early prostate cancer, but the cohort study discussed above shows that ten-year disease-specific survival rates for patients treated this way is similar to those treated with watchful waiting for well and moderately differentiated prostate cancer, but higher for those with poorly differentiated tumours [48] **(III/B)**.

The relatively new treatment of brachytherapy for men with localised prostate cancer does not have any RCTs to support it, but observational studies have shown good survival rates for patients treated this way [53, 54].

Harm of screening and of treatments

The harm of entering asymptomatic patients into a screening programme mostly encompasses the harm of the screening tests and pathway, but the harm caused by any of the treatments which patients might subsequently undergo also need to be considered.

Screening tests

The preliminary screening tests themselves, PSA and DRE, are likely to be acceptable to the vast majority of the population, and have no long-term harm in themselves. However, the anxiety that they and the screening process as a whole may generate is unknown, but may well be significant. The subsequent investigation of transrectal ultrasound and biopsy does have morbidity, though major complications requiring hospitalisation are rare. Pain or discomfort from the biopsy is common, with up to 30% of patients reporting the procedure as being significantly painful [55], although for patients under 60 years this may be as high as 78% [56]. Minor immediate complications are common, consisting of rectal bleeding (2.1%), mild haematuria (62%), haemospermia (9.8%), and persistent dysuria (7.2%) in patients undergoing their first biopsy. More serious complications included urinary tract infection (10.9%), urinary retention (2.7%), and vasovagal episodes (2.8%) [56].

Harm of treatment

The radical treatments on offer to patients diagnosed with early prostate cancer do come at a cost in terms of morbidity from the treatment received. Radical prostatectomy is associated with surgical mortality, though this is now generally below 1%. Other acute complications are relatively minor, and total 8% in one recent series of over 300 patients [57], but longer-term problems include urinary incontinence and erectile dysfunction. Radical radiotherapy has early side effects which include tenesmus, diarrhoea and general fatigue, but these are usually only temporary. Later side effects include intestinal inflammation and bleeding, urinary incontinence and impotence. Brachytherapy may lead to a worsening of or development of lower urinary tract symptoms, urinary retention, incontinence, erectile dysfunction and intestinal inflammatory problems.

Erectile dysfunction

One meta-analysis of 40 studies examined the rates of erectile dysfunction after radical prostatectomy (RP) and external beam radiotherapy (EBRT), and found a 42% chance of maintaining erectile function after RP, and 69% chance after EBRT [58]. In a good quality questionnaire-based study that asked patients about their sexual function pre- and post-treatment, erectile dysfunction increased from 32% at baseline to 93% at 12 months for those undergoing RP, and from 45% to 67% for those who had EBRT [59]. Furthermore, nerve-sparing RP resulted in the same amount of erectile dysfunction as those who had a non-nerve-sparing procedure. However, potency rates as high as 86% 18 months after a nerve-sparing RP, with or without the use of sildenafil, have been reported [60]. Fowler *et al* reported on the results of 621 patients who underwent radical radiotherapy and 373 who had radical prostatectomy and erectile dysfunction was higher in the RP group (56% vs 23%) [61]. Brachytherapy has relatively low rates of erectile dysfunction, with potency rates commonly reported at between 50%-86% [62, 63].

Urinary incontinence

Fowler *et al* reported on the results of 621 patients who underwent radical radiotherapy and 373 who had radical prostatectomy. Urinary incontinence was higher in the surgical group (32% vs 7%) [61]. In the same questionnaire-based study previously mentioned [59], urinary incontinence, defined as the percentage of patients wearing pads, increased from 3% at baseline to 35% at 12 months for RP patients, and from 1% at baseline to 5% for EBRT patients. In a small study of 64 patients with localised prostate cancer who underwent RP, continence rates of 93% at 18 months have been reported in one specialised centre [60]. Urinary incontinence is rare in those who are treated with brachytherapy, and may be as low as 1% in those who have not had a TURP [64, 65]. However, patients treated with brachytherapy may develop urinary retention, and while some report the incidence is as low as 5% [65], it may be higher and has been reported at 15% in one larger study [66].

GI symptoms

In the same questionnaire-based study previously mentioned [59], bowel symptoms defined as the percentage of patients with bowel urgency or tenderness, decreased from 7% at baseline to 6% at 12 months for RP patients, and increased from 1% at baseline to 19% for EBRT patients. Other studies which have compared bowel function in men who had undergone EBRT compared to controls showed that between 10% and 25% more men reported marked bowel problems, most commonly symptoms attributable to rectal inflammation [67, 68]. Radiation proctitis has been reported to occur in between 1%-39% in patients undergoing brachytherapy, but this is usually mild in most patients [69].

There is only one randomised controlled study looking at quality of life and the harm of treatment for localised prostate cancer compared to controls (watchful waiting). In this study, symptom and quality of life questionnaires were returned from 166 of 189 men who underwent radical prostatectomy, and 160 of 187 men assigned to watchful waiting at a mean of four years after randomisation. Erectile dysfunction was more common in the RP group (80% vs 45%), as was urinary leakage (49% vs 21%), while urinary obstruction was less common (28% vs 44%). However, there was no difference in subjective quality of life, anxiety or depression [70] **(Ib/A)**.

Cost-effectiveness of screening

It is very difficult to estimate the cost-effectiveness of screening for prostate cancer given all the uncertainties surrounding potential benefits and harm, but some authors have attempted to calculate these. One author in the USA estimated that the costs of a screening and treatment programme for a single year would be between $17.6 billion and $25.7 billion, at prices from over ten years ago [71].

In 1993, a decision analysis of alternative treatment strategies modelled the benefit of treatment as a reduction in chance of death or morbidity from metastatic disease, and offset these against the risks of treatment-related morbidity and mortality. The findings suggested that patients with well differentiated tumours had limited benefit, but for those with moderately or poorly differentiated tumours, screening and early radical treatment may offer as much as 3.5 years increase in quality-adjusted life expectancy [72]. A further conclusion was that treatment for men older than 70 years appears to be harmful.

Cost per life-year saved is often a way in which the cost-effectiveness of screening is calculated, and using favourable assumptions in a man aged 65, without adjustment for iatrogenic morbidity, this figure has been calculated at approximately $15,000. However, using less favourable assumptions, the cost may be as high as $100,000 [73].

In summary, screening may be cost-effective for patients under 70 years, if favourable assumptions are made about the efficacy of screening.

Effectiveness of screening programmes

There is very little good evidence currently on the effectiveness of screening programmes, but the data from two large ongoing studies should provide the answers we seek, but not for several years. The European Randomised Study of Screening for Prostate Cancer (ERSPC) study started in 1994, and is randomising 190,000 men aged 50-75 to screening with DRE, PSA and TRUS, or usual care. The "Prostate, Lung, Colorectal and Ovary" (PCLO) trial started in 1995, and it is randomising 74,000 men aged 60-74 to annual screening for four years with DRE and PSA, and comparing this to standard care as well.

The only randomised trial performed to date by Labrie et al studied 46,193 men; 30,956 men were randomised to screening using PSA (upper limit of normal 3.0ng/ml) and DRE, and the rest to observation. TRUS was performed only if PSA and/or DRE were abnormal, and a biopsy then performed if PSA was high or a hypoechoic lesion was seen. In this study, of the 30,956 men who were randomised to screening, 7,155 actually underwent screening while 23,801 did not. Of the 15,237 who were randomised to observation, 982 actually underwent screening while 14,255 did not. One hundred and thirty-seven deaths were noted among the 38,056

men who did not undergo screening compared to only five deaths among the 8,137 men who underwent screening. Thus, prostate cancer death rates in the screened and unscreened populations during the eight-year period were 15 and 48.7 per 100,000 man years, a figure which gives a 69% decrease in deaths from prostate cancer in favour of screening and early treatment. However, using an intention-to-treat analysis based upon the study arm to which the individual was originally randomised, there was no difference in mortality, there were 73 deaths among the 15,237 men (4.8 per 100,000) who were randomised to observation compared to 140 deaths among the 31,300 randomised to screening (4.6 per 100,000). Thus, because of non-compliance, this study does not answer the question whether early detection with PSA and DRE will reduce prostate cancer mortality [74].

Three case control studies provide conflicting information on the efficacy of screening for prostate cancer using DRE [12, 75, 76]. Only one of them found that having had a DRE may protect men from advanced prostate cancer or from dying from prostate cancer [12], while the other two found no such benefit [75, 76]. While the reason for the differences between these studies is not clear, all three were small, and all three have the major problem that they are unable to distinguish between diagnostic and screening DRE. Furthermore, there has been criticism of the only study with positive findings [77].

Ecologic data have shown that the incidence of prostate cancer in the USA rose dramatically during the early 1990s after the introduction of PSA testing, and then subsequently decreased as did mortality from the disease [78]. This has been directly attributed to introduction of PSA screening by some [79]. However, there are a number of factors which suggest that this may not be the case [80]. Data from the Tyrol longitudinal cohort study supports the view that screening leads to decreased mortality from prostate cancer [81], whereas that from another suggests that there is no difference in two populations of patients subjected to different levels of screening for prostate cancer [82]. The two cohorts of patient in this latter study were elderly (65-79 years) however, and this may be the reason for the lack of benefit found with screening in this paper.

Thus, current evidence from the single randomised controlled study, case control studies and observational data, does not provide sufficient evidence that screening for prostate cancer can affect mortality from prostate cancer, and we must await the data from the two large randomised controlled studies which are ongoing **(IV/C)**.

Conclusions

Wilson and Jungner set out the criteria for the implementation of a screening programme over 30 years ago, and while not perfect, these criteria are still applicable today when considering whether we should screen for a disease. Thus, whilst we can agree that prostate cancer is an important health problem, that we understand the natural history of the disease to an increasing extent, that we do have a suitable screening test that is acceptable to the general population, we currently have some evidence that radical treatment is more effective than watchful waiting. We also have evidence that the screening process and the subsequent treatments can cause harm. On this basis, the criteria set out by Wilson and Jungner have not been met to date, and lack of any good evidence that screening is worthwhile from randomised controlled trials would support this view.

The results of the PCLO and ERSPC studies are eagerly awaited however, with the hope that the findings will still be relevant to current practice when they are published. The danger is that improvements in the screening tests, or in identifying which tumours are likely to shorten their carrier's life, or in treatments for the disease, may render such findings of these studies non-applicable when they are finally available. At least, whatever the situation is at this point, our understanding of the disease and its treatment will have improved, which will benefit our patients.

Recommendations	Evidence level
◆ Prostate cancer poses an important health problem.	IV/C
◆ PSA testing is a sensitive and specific test for the diagnosis for early prostate cancer.	IIb/B
◆ PSA testing can detect prostate cancer at an earlier clinical stage.	III/B
◆ Treatment of early prostate cancer by radical prostatectomy decreases cancer-related mortality, but has not yet been shown to significantly affect overall mortality.	Ib/A
◆ Disease-specific survival is higher for men with moderately and poorly differentiated tumours who undergo radical prostatectomy compared to both radiotherapy and watchful waiting, and higher in men with poorly differentiated tumours undergoing radical radiotherapy compared to watchful waiting.	III/B
◆ Treatment of early prostate cancer causes morbidity.	Ib/A
◆ There is no good evidence that screening for prostate cancer improves mortality.	IV/C

Chapter 13

References

1. Wilson JMG, Jungner G. Principles and practice of screening for disease. Public Health Paper Number 34. World Health Organisation, Geneva, 1968.
2. Frankel S, Davey Smith G, Donovan J, Neal D. Screening for prostate cancer. *Lancet* 2003; 361: 1122-28.
3. Office for National Statistics. Cancer trends in England and Wales 1950-1999. Stationery Office, London, 1999.
4. American Cancer Society. Cancer Facts and Figures 2003. Available at: www.cancer.org.
5. Whitmore WF Jnr. Localised prostate cancer: management and detection issues. *Lancet* 1994; 343: 1263-67.
6. Johansson JE, Adami HO, Andersson SO, *et al.* High 10- year survival rate in patients with early untreated prostate cancer. *JAMA* 1992; 267(16): 2191-96.
7. Albertsen PC, Hanley JA, Gleason DF, Barry MJ. Competing risk analysis of men aged 55-74 years at diagnosis managed conservatively for clinically localised prostate cancer. *JAMA* 1998; 280: 975-80.
8. McNeal JE. Origin and development of carcinoma in the prostate. *Cancer* 1969; 23(1): 24-34.
9. McNeal JE, Bostwick DG, Kindrachuk RA, *et al.* Patterns of progression in prostate cancer. *Lancet* 1986; 1(8472): 60-3.
10. Smith DS, Catalona WJ. Interexaminer variability of digital rectal examination in detecting prostate cancer. *Urology* 1995; 45: 70-74.
11. Catalona WJ, Rirchie JP, Ahmann FR, *et al.* Comparison of DRE and serum PSA in the early detection of prostate cancer: results of a multi-centre clinical trial of 6,630 men. *J Urol* 1994; 151: 1283-90.
12. Jacobsen SJ, Bergstralh EJ, Katusic SK, *et al.* Screening digital rectal examination and prostate cancer mortality: a population-based case-control study. *Urology* 1998; 52(2): 173-179.
13. Mettlin C, Lee F, Drago J, Murphy GP. The American Cancer Society National Prostate Cancer detection project. Findings on detection of early prostate cancer in 2,425 men. *Cancer* 1991; 67 (12): 2949-58.
14. Gustafsson O, Norming U, Almgard LE, *et al.* Diagnostic methods in the detection of prostate cancer: a study of a randomly selected population of 2,400 men. *J Urol* 1992; 148: 1827-31.
15. Gann PH, Hennekens CH, Stampfer MJ. A prospective evaluation of plasma prostate-specific antigen for detection of prostatic cancer. *J Urol* 1995; 273: 289-94.
16. Mettlin C, Murphy GP, Babaian RJ, *et al.* The results of a five-year early prostate cancer detection intervention. Investigators of the American Cancer Society National Cancer Detection Project. *Cancer* 1996; 77: 150-9.
17. Schroder FH, van der Cruijsen-Koeter I, de Koning HJ, *et al.* Prostate cancer detection at low prostate specific antigen. *J Urol* 2000; 163: 806-12.
18. Catalona WJ, Miller DR, Kavoussi LR. Intermediate-term survival results in clinically understaged prostate cancer patients following radical prostatectomy. *J Urol* 1998; 140: 540-3.
19. Catalona WJ, Smith DS, Ratliff TL, *et al.* Measurement of prostate specific antigen in serum as a screening test for prostate cancer. *N Engl J Med* 1991; 324(17): 1156-61.
20. Brawer MK. Prostate-specific antigen: current status. *CA Cancer J Clin* 1999; 49(5): 264-281.
21. McLaughlin AP, Saltzstein SL, McCullough DL, *et al.* Prostatic carcinoma: incidence and location of unsuspected lymphatic metastases. *J Urol* 1976; 115: 89-94.
22. Thompson IM, Ernst JJ, Gangai MP, *et al.* Adenocarcinoma of the prostate: results of routine urological screening. *J Urol* 1984; 132: 690-692.
23. Partin AW, Kattan MW, Subong ENP, *et al.* Combination of prostate-specific antigen, clinical stage, and Gleason score to predict pathological stage of localized prostate cancer: a multi-institutional update. *JAMA* 1997; 277(18): 1445-1451.
24. Smith DS, Catalona WJ, Herschman JD. Longitudinal screening for prostate cancer with prostate specific antigen. *JAMA* 1996; 276(16): 1309-1315.
25. Rietbergen JB, Hoedemaeker RF, Kruger AE, *et al.* The changing pattern of prostate cancer at the time of diagnosis: characteristics of screen detected prostate cancer in a population-based screening study. *J Urol* 1999; 161(4): 1192-8.
26. Maatenen L, Auvinen A, Stenman U-H, *et al.* European randomised study of prostate cancer screening: first year results of the Finnish trial. *Br J Cancer* 1999; 79: 1210-14.
27. Cooner WH, Mosley BR, Rutherford CL Jr, *et al.* Prostate cancer detection in a clinical urological practice by ultrasonography, digital rectal examination and prostate specific antigen. *J Urol* 1990; 143: 1146-52.
28. Hammerer P, Huland H. Systematic sextant biopsies in 651 patients referred for prostate evaluation. *J Urol* 1994; 151: 99-102.
29. Schroder FH, van der Maas P, Beemsterboer P, *et al.* Evaluation of the digital rectal examination as a screening test for prostate cancer. Rotterdam section of the European Randomized Study of Screening for Prostate Cancer. *J Natl Cancer Inst* 1998; 90: 1817-23.
30. Catalona WJ, Smith DS, Ornstein DK. Prostate cancer detection in men with serum PSA concentrations of 2.6 to 4.0ng/ml and benign prostatic examination: enhancement of specificity with free PSA measurements. *JAMA* 1997; 277: 1452-55.
31. Labrie F, Dupont A, Suburu R, *et al.* Serum prostate specific antigen as pre-screening for prostate cancer. *J Urol* 1992; 147: 846-51.
32. Carter HB, Pearson JD, Metter EJ, *et al.* Longitudinal evaluation of prostate-specific antigen levels in men with and without prostate disease. *JAMA* 1992; 267(16): 2215-2220.
33. Brawer MK, Beatie J, Wener MH, *et al.* Screening for prostatic carcinoma with prostate specific antigen: results of the second year. *J Urol* 1993; 150(1): 106-109.
34. Benson MC, Whang IS, Pantuck A, *et al.* Prostate specific antigen density: a means of distinguishing benign prostatic hypertrophy and prostate cancer. *J Urol* 1992; 147(3 pt 2): 815-816.

Chapter 13

35. Seaman E., Whang IS, Olsson CA, *et al.* PSA density (PSAD). Role in patient evaluation and management. *Urol Clin N Am* 1993; 20: 653-63.

36. Catalona WJ, Ritchie JP, deKernion JB, *et al.* Comparison of prostate specific antigen concentration versus prostate specific antigen density in the early detection of prostate cancer: receiver operating characteristic curves. *J Urol* 1994; 152: 2031-6.

37. Kalish J, Cooner WH, Graham SD. Serum PSA adjusted for volume of transition zone (PSAT) is more accurate than PSA adjusted for total gland volume (PSAD) in detecting adenocarcinoma of the prostate. *Urology* 1994; 43: 601-606.

38. Djavan B, Zlotta AR, Remzi M, *et al.* Total and transition zone prostate volume and age: how do they affect the utility of PSA-based diagnostic parameters for early prostate cancer detection? *Urology* 1999; 54(5): 846-52.

39. Oesterling JE, Jacobsen SJ, Chute CG, *et al.* Serum prostate-specific antigen in a community-based population of healthy men: establishment of age-specific reference ranges. *JAMA* 1993; 270(7): 860-4.

40. Reissigl A, Pointner J, Horninger W, *et al.* Comparison of different prostate specific antigen cutpoints for early detection of prostate cancer: results of a large screening study. *Urology* 1995: 46(5): 662-5.

41. Stenman UH, Leinonen J, Alftham H, *et al.* A complex between prostate-specific antigen and a1-antichymotripsin is the major form of prostate-specific antigen in serum of patients with prostatic cancer: assay of the complex improves clinical sensitivity for cancer. *Cancer Res* 1991; 51: 222-6.

42. Lilja H, Christensson A., Dahlen U, *et al.* Prostate specific antigen in the serum occurs predominantly in complex with alpha-1 antichymotrypsin. *Clin Chem* 1991; 37(9): 1618-25.

43. Polascik TJ, Oesterling JE, Partin AW. Prostate Specific Antigen: a decade of discovery - what we have learned and where we are going. *J Urol* 1999, 162: 293-6.

44. Catalona WJ, Partin AW, Slawin KM, *et al.* A multicentre clinical trial evaluation of free PSA in the differentiation of prostate cancer from benign disease. *J Urol* 1997; 157: 111-abstract 434.

45. Waterhouse RL, Resnick MI. The use of transrectal prostatic ultrasonography in the evaluation of patients with prostatic carcinoma. *J Urol* 1989; 141(2): 233-239.

46. Klein EA, Kupelian PA. Localised prostate cancer: radiation or surgery. *Urol Clin N Am* 2003; 30: 315-30.

47. Holmberg L, Bill-Axelson A, Helgesen F, *et al.* Scandinavian Prostatic Cancer Group Study Number 4. A randomized trial comparing radical prostatectomy with watchful waiting in early prostate cancer. *N Engl J Med* 2002; 347(11): 781-9.

48. Lu-Yao GL, Yao SL. Population-based study of long-term survival in patients with clinically localised prostate cancer. *Lancet* 1997; 349: 906-10.

49. Kupelian PA, Elshaik M, Reddy CA, *et al.* Comparison of the efficacy of local therapies for localised prostate cancer in the Prostate-Specific Antigen era: a large single institution experience with radical prostatectomy and external-beam radiotherapy. *J Clin Oncol* 2002; 20: 3376-85.

50. Pollack A, Zagars GK, Starkschall G, *et al.* Prostate cancer radiation dose response: results of the M.D. Anderson phase III randomized trial. *Int J Radiat Oncol Biol Phys* 2002; 53(5): 1097-105.

51. Jhaveri FM, Zippe CD, Klein EA, *et al.* Biochemical failure does not predict overall survival after radical prostatectomy for localised prostate cancer: 10-year results. *Urology* 1999; 54: 884-90.

52. Kupelain P, Buchsbaum J, Patel C, *et al.* Impact of biochemical failure as a predictor of overall survival in men with localised prostate cancer treated with radiotherapy. *Int J Radiat Oncol Biol Phys* 2002; 52: 704-11.

53. Hochstetler JA, Kreder KJ, Brown CK, Loening SA. Survival of patients with localised prostate cancer treated with percutaneous transperineal placement of radioactive gold seeds: stages A2, B and C. *Prostate* 1995; 26: 316-24.

54. Schellhammer PF, Moriarty R, Bostwick D, *et al.* Fifteen-year minimum follow-up of a prostate brachytherapy series: comparing the past with the present. *Urology* 2000; 56: 436-9.

55. Clemens R, Aideyan OU, Griffiths GJ, *et al.* Side effects and patients' acceptability of transrectal biopsy of the prostate. *Clin Radiol* 1993; 47: 125-6.

56. Djavan B, Waldert M, Zlotta A. Safety and morbidity of first and repeat transrectal ultrasound-guided prostate needle biopsies: results of a prospective European prostate cancer detection study. *J Urol* 2001; 166: 856-60.

57. Ng CS, Klein EA. Acute complications after radical retropubic prostatectomy. *The Prostate Journal* 2000; 2: 22-6.

58. Robinson JW, Dufour MS, Fung TS. Erectile functioning of men treated for prostate carcinoma. *Cancer* 1997; 79: 538-44.

59. Talcott JA, Rieker P, Clark JA, *et al.* Patient-reported symptoms after primary therapy for early prostate cancer: results of a prospective cohort study. *J Clin Oncol* 1998; 16: 275-83.

60. Walsh PC, Marschke P, Ricker D, Burnett AL. Patient-reported urinary continence and sexual function after anatomic radical prostatectomy. *Urology* 2000; 55(1): 58-61.

61. Fowler FJ, Barry MJ, Lu-Yao G, *et al.* Outcomes of external beam radiation treatment for prostate cancer: a study of medicare beneficiaries in three surveillance epidemiology and end results areas. *J Clin Oncol* 1996; 14: 2258-65.

62. Wallner K, Roy J, Harrisson L. Tumour control and morbidity following transperineal iodine 125 implantation for stage T1/T2 prostatic carcinoma. *J Clin Oncol* 1996; 14: 449-53.

63. Potters L, Torre T, Fearn PA, *et al.* Potency after permanent prostate brachytherapy for localized prostate cancer. *Int J Radiat Oncol Biol Phys* 2001; 50(5): 1235-42.

64. Ragde H, Blasko JC, Grimm PD, *et al.* Brachytherapy for clinically localised prostate cancer: results at 7 and 8 years follow-up. *Seminars in Surg Oncol* 1997; 13: 438-43.

65. Terk MD, Stock RG, Stone NN. Identification of patients at increased risk for prolonged urinary retention following radioactive seed implantation of the prostate. *J Urol* 1998; 160: 1379-82.

66. Bucci J, Morris WJ, Keyes M, *et al.* Predictive factors of urinary retention following prostate brachytherapy. *Int J Radiat Oncol Biol Phys* 2002; 53(1): 91-8.

Chapter 13

67. Widmark A, Fransson P, Tavelin B. Self-assessment questionnaire for evaluating urinary and intestinal late side effects after pelvic radiotherapy in patients with prostate cancer compared with an age matched population. *Cancer* 1994; 74: 2520-32.

68. Litwin MS. Health related quality of life after treatment for localised prostate cancer. *Cancer* 1995; 75: 2000-03.

69. Stone NN, Stock RG. Practical considerations in permanent brachytherapy for localised adenocarcinoma of the prostate. *Urol Clin N Am* 2003: 30: 351-62.

70. Steineck G, Helgesen F, Adolfsson J, *et al*. Quality of life after radical prostatectomy or watchful waiting. *N Engl J Med* 2002; 347(11): 790-6.

71. Lubke WL, Optenberg SA, Thompson IM. Analysis of the first-year cost of a prostate cancer screening and treatment program in the United States. *J Natl Cancer Inst* 1994; 86(23): 1790-2.

72. Fleming C, Wasson JH, Albertsen PC, *et al*. A decision analysis of alternative treatment strategies for clinically localised prostate cancer. Prostate Patients Outcomes Research Team. *JAMA* 1993; 269: 2650-8.

73. Barry MJ, Fleming C, Coley CM, *et al*. Should Medicare provide reimbursement for prostate-specific antigen testing for early detection of prostate cancer? Part IV: estimating the risks and benefits of an early detection program. *Urology* 1995; 46: 445-61.

74. Labrie F, Candas B, Dupont A, *et al*. Screening decreases prostate cancer death: first analysis of the 1988 Quebec prospective randomized controlled trial. *The Prostate* 1999; 38(2): 83-91.

75. Friedman GD, Hiatt RA, Queensbury CP Jr, *et al*. Case-control study of screening for prostate cancer by digital rectal examination. *Lancet* 1991; 337: 1526-9.

76. Richert-Boe KE, Humphrey LL, Glass AG, *et al*. Screening digital rectal examination and prostate cancer mortality: a case control study. *J Med Screen* 1998; 5: 99-103.

77. Weiss NS, Friedman GD. Digital rectal examination and mortality from prostate cancer. *Urology* 1999; 53(4): 863-4.

78. Hankey BF, Feuer EJ, Clegg LX, *et al*. Cancer surveillance series: interpreting trends in prostate cancer. Part 1: evidence of the effects of screening in recent prostate cancer incidence, mortality and survival rates. *J Natl Cancer Inst* 1999; 91: 1017-24.

79. Farkas A, Schneider D, Perrotti M, *et al*. National trends in the epidemiology of prostate cancer 1973-94: evidence for the effectiveness of prostate-specific antigen screening. *Urology* 1998; 52(3): 444-8.

80. Harris R, Lohr KN. Screening for prostate cancer: an update of the evidence for the U.S Preventative Services Taskforce. *Ann Int Medicine* 2002; 137(11): 917-29.

81. Bartsch G, Horninger W, Klocker H, *et al*. Prostate cancer mortality after introduction of prostate-specific antigen mass screening in the federal state of Tyrol, Austria. *Urology* 2001; 58: 417-24.

82. Lu-Yao G, Albertsen PC, Stanford JL, *et al*. Natural experiment examining impact of aggressive screening and treatment on prostate cancer mortality in two fixed cohorts from Seattle area and Connecticut. *BMJ* 2002; 325: 740-3.

Chapter 13

Chapter 14

Is radiological imaging worthwhile in patients with clinically localised prostate cancer?

Chris Dawson BSc MS FRCS

Consultant Urologist

EDITH CAVELL HOSPITAL, PETERBOROUGH, UK

Introduction

The staging of prostate cancer is an important issue, because much depends upon the correct assessment of the stage of the disease. In general, locally confined prostate cancer is amenable to treatment with either watchful waiting, radical prostatectomy, radiotherapy (either conformal radiotherapy, or brachytherapy), or hormones. Once the disease has become locally advanced, the treatment options may be decreased since many surgeons would consider radical surgery to be an inappropriate option.

The role of imaging in the staging of prostate cancer remains controversial. This chapter sets out to review the available imaging options and to ascertain the levels of evidence (where appropriate) to substantiate their usage.

Methodology

A Medline search was employed to gather evidence, using the search terms "prostate cancer", "localised", "imaging", "CT", "MRI".

According to the TNM Classification of tumours [1], localised prostate cancer by definition must be either pT1 or pT2 disease. Localised disease must also be free of nodal metastasis (N0) or distant metastasis (M0).

What are the available methods for staging prostate cancer?

A number of methods are available for staging prostate cancer. Digital rectal examination (DRE) is used both for diagnostic purposes and to assign a clinical stage to the tumour once confirmed histologically. Studies have shown that DRE is not a very sensitive test and may understage the level of disease in up to 50% of cases [2-4]. In one study, T2 tumours (localised) could only be distinguished from T3 tumours (locally advanced) in 69% of cases [5]. In another study, Narayan *et al* found that 56% of patients with T3 disease on DRE had organ-confined disease at final histological analysis [6] **(IIa/B)**.

Prostate specific antigen (PSA) is routinely used as an aid to diagnosis in men presenting with lower urinary tract symptoms (LUTS). The use of PSA as a

Chapter 14

screening tool in asymptomatic men remains the subject of controversy and will not be considered further in this article. Earlier studies on PSA have revealed figures for sensitivity ranging from 46%-90% and specificity from 59%-72%. Figures for overall accuracy range from 64%-91% [7].

For this reason, the use of DRE and PSA, either alone or in combination, is not considered sufficiently accurate to stage prostate cancer.

The remainder of this chapter will consider the available imaging techniques including transrectal ultrasonography (TRUS), computerised tomography (CT), magnetic resonance imaging (MRI) and its variants, isotope scans, and other more recent developments.

Transrectal ultrasound scanning (TRUS) in locally confined prostate cancer

The introduction of TRUS in the 1980s led to a significant advance in the diagnostic potential for prostate cancer. Early enthusiasm that TRUS would lead to improved staging of prostate cancer has, however, proved unfounded.

Initially, it was felt that prostate cancer would appear as hypoechoic areas on the scans - it is now known that prostate cancers may appear as hypo-, hyper-, or iso-echoic areas [8-9]. For this reason, TRUS is also not very effective at detecting the extent of cancer within the prostate.

Whilst early studies appeared to show high sensitivity for the prediction of capsular involvement [10], it now appears that TRUS is no better at detecting local extension of prostate cancer than DRE [11] **(III/B)**.

Most urologists now feel that the main advantage of TRUS is to allow for proper placement of the biopsy needle and to allow for adequate sampling of the whole of the prostate gland.

The role of computerised tomography in localised prostate cancer

CT scanning is now widely available in most radiology departments. However, studies have shown that the resolution of CT is too low to be able to distinguish abnormalities within the prostate gland, the state of the capsule, or the presence or absence of disease outside of the prostate gland [12-15]. In one study, CT scanning prior to radical prostatectomy was only able to predict extracapsular spread or seminal vesicle invasion in 10% of cases [16] **(III/B)**.

CT may have a role in evaluating the state of the lymph nodes alongside the prostate gland in patients considered suitable for radical surgery or radiotherapy. The use of Partin's tables [17] or Kattan's nomograms [18] will help decide which patients are at risk of nodal metastasis. Caution needs to be observed in reporting CT scans in such patients. Enlarged nodes due to inflammation may give rise to false positive results and mean that patients are not considered for radical treatment. Conversely, metastasis may be present in small nodes with microscopic involvement. Such nodes will usually be beyond the limit of detection of CT and give rise to false negative results [19].

The role of magnetic resonance imaging in localised prostate cancer

MRI scanning began with the use of the body coil, which generates a large field of view. The endorectal coil, which was first developed in 1988, has a much higher signal to noise ratio and thus allows for prostatic images with much higher resolution [20,21]. With improvements in technique, the maximal resolution of images is approximately 3mm [19]. Other factors which affect the quality of images include the strength of the magnetic field used and the type of pulse sequence employed [22].

MRI provides high quality images of the prostate and can differentiate well between the different anatomic zones of the prostate [22,23]. The appearance of the prostate is different on T1 weighted and T2 weighted images. Little difference is seen between the different anatomic zones on T1 weighted images, but on T2 weighted images, the peripheral zone appears as a "hyperintense" zone compared to the central and transitional zones which remain low in signal intensity [24,25].

Prostate cancer may appear as any one of the following patterns:

- A region of low signal intensity on both T1 and T2 weighted images in the peripheral zone of the prostate [24-27].
- Multiple areas of low signal on T2 weighted images [24].
- A diffuse abnormality of low signal throughout the peripheral zone of the prostate [24].

Care should be taken when interpreting the MRI images of the prostate gland. Areas of haemorrhage following prostate biopsy may also appear as low signal lesions on T2 weighted images, and some authors recommend that MRI should be deferred after prostate biopsy for at least three weeks [26,27]. Prostatitis may cause a similar finding, and prior radiation therapy or treatment with hormones can decrease the signal intensity of the peripheral zone on T2 weighted images [21].

The main purpose of MRI scanning in patients suspected clinically to have locally confined prostate cancer, is to establish whether extracapsular spread or distant metastasis has occurred. Such a finding may preclude intervention with radical therapy. If normal hyperintense tissue is seen between the tumour and the capsule on T2 weighted images, this would suggest that the tumour is confined to the prostate [20]. Signs of extracapsular penetration include an irregular gland or irregularity of the capsule, or obvious disruption of the capsule. More distant spread may appear as a low signal "stranding" appearance in the periprostatic fat, or loss of the fat plane between the prostate and rectum [26].

Various studies have shown that MRI has a sensitivity ranging from 51%-95%, a specificity from 67%-100%, and an overall accuracy from 47%-88% [20,24].

When is an MRI of the prostate useful in prostate cancer?

Non-palpable prostate cancer

Werner-Wasik *et al* investigated the use of both transrectal ultrasound (TRUS) and MRI in 291 men with clinically non-palpable prostate cancer [28]. An analysis of the TRUS and MRI results revealed that only 12% of the men with non-palpable tumours had normal TRUS and MRI, and thus could be truly classified as stage T1c according to the TNM classification (i.e. non-palpable, not visible on imaging, PSA-detected cancer). Despite this, there was no significant difference in the PSA levels, Gleason scores, and probability of the disease being bilateral compared to unilateral, between this group and patients with non-palpable prostate cancer visible on imaging. In view of this, there may be little use in upstaging T1c disease to T2 disease (but still non-palpable) on the basis of imaging results.

Clinically localised prostate cancer

D'Amico *et al* reported on the use of endorectal MRI for predicting time to PSA failure after radical prostatectomy in 1025 consecutive patients [29]. Having allowed for PSA, Gleason score, clinical T stage, and the percent of positive biopsies, they found that endorectal MRI added useful information in only 19% of cases. An earlier study by the same authors of 445 patients undergoing radical prostatectomy attempted to correlate the degree of agreement of endorectal MRI with the pathological findings of extracapsular extension and seminal vesicle invasion [30]. As the PSA level and biopsy Gleason score increased pre-operatively, there was less correlation between the pathological findings and the endorectal scans, presumably, as the authors stated, because of microscopic extracapsular involvement leading to false negative MRI scans. Endorectal MRI scans had some value in predicting PSA failure in those patients who could not be assigned to a high or low risk group for PSA failure by virtue of their pre-operative parameters.

Chapter 14

Differentiating T2 and T3 prostate cancer

There is increasing evidence that MRI scanning has a use in differentiating palpable, but locally confined, (T2) prostate cancer from locally advanced (T3) prostate cancer. D'Amico et al looked at the use of endorectal MRI in patients with clinical stage T1 or T2 disease, a PSA of between 10 and 20ng/ml, and a Gleason score of 7 or less [31]. In their study, endorectal MRI predicted extracapsular penetration and seminal vesicle involvement with an accuracy of 84%. Endorectal MRI would have improved the organ-confined disease rate from 32% to 61%, and significantly improved the PSA failure rate **(III/B)**.

Other studies have reported that endorectal coil MRI has an accuracy between 64% and 85% for correctly predicting stage T3 prostate cancer [19].

Predicting lymph node involvement

The removal of lymph nodes along the obturator chains during radical prostatectomy is now fairly routine. The finding of cancer in the lymph nodes equates to incurable disease and most surgeons would not proceed with radical prostatectomy [32]. To a large extent, the likelihood of lymph node metastasis can be obtained from Kattan's nomograms[18] according to the pre-operative PSA, clinical stage, and biopsy Gleason score.

Although MRI is superior to CT in visualising intraprostatic architecture and local disease extension, it does not appear to offer any advantages in evaluation of the local lymph nodes [32]. The only reliable sign of lymph node metastasis on MRI is enlargement of the node, as there is no specific change in signal intensity. For this reason, MRI is unable to detect metastatic tumour in lymph nodes of normal size [33]. MRI appears to have a sensitivity and specificity for lymph node involvement of 42% and 98% respectively [34], and the poor predictive value of MRI suggests that MRI is not useful in detecting pelvic node metastasis prior to surgery [35].

Several authors have reviewed the literature to try and reach a consensus about the place of MRI in prostate cancer staging. Jager et al in 2000 used a "decision analytic approach" having reviewed the available literature at that time [36]. They found that patients at intermediate risk of extracapsular penetration or seminal vesicle disease (i.e. PSA between 10-20ng/ml and Gleason score of 5-7), benefited from having MRI scanning. The quality adjusted life years (QALYs) after radical prostatectomy were similar whether or not MRI scanning was used for staging purposes. Overall, however, they concluded that the literature did not support the use of routine MRI scanning as a pre-operative investigation for men with prostate cancer.

A similar analytical approach was taken by Wolf et al in their 1995 paper [37]. They retrospectively reviewed 174 patients who had undergone radical prostatectomy and been found histologically to have metastatic lymph node involvement. They reported a sensitivity for detecting nodal metastasis of only 25% and felt that MRI scanning solely to detect lymph node spread was not routinely indicated, although there was justification for patients at high risk for nodal metastasis.

Engelbrecht et al produced a meta-analysis in 2002 on MRI scanning in the local staging of prostate cancer, looking at articles published between 1984 and 2000 [38]. They were unable to explain the large variation in performance of MRI scanning in local staging. What is clear from their analysis is the wide discrepancy in the criteria used for the definition of extracapsular spread, and the large number of missing data on patient characteristics in the published studies. They conclude that future studies should improve the quality of reporting and that caution should be applied to the interpretation of studies with small sample sizes in which the staging performance may be higher than expected.

Isotope bone scanning in localised prostate cancer

Isotope, or radionuclide bone scanning is used to detect bone metastasis in patients with newly diagnosed prostate cancer. Such deposits, in their early stages, can be present without symptoms.

Although isotope bone scanning remains the most accurate form of imaging for this purpose [39], not all newly diagnosed patients require a bone scan. Chybowski *et al* found no evidence of bone metastasis in 209 patients with a PSA of 10ng/ml or less, and only one patient out of 306 with a PSA of 20ng/ml or less had bone metastases [40] **(III/B)**. Similar results were reported by Oesterling *et al* who found a positive bone scan rate of 0.8% in patients with a PSA less than 20ng/ml. They found no positive bone scans in patients with a PSA of 8ng/ml or less [41].

New developments in imaging

Single photon computerised tomography (SPECT)

SPECT is a type of CT scan in which radio-labelled compounds are used to produce tomographic images of the distribution of radioactivity *in vivo* [42]. Although more rapid than conventional CT imaging there appears to be little data on its potential for use in clinically localised prostate cancer.

Magnetic resonance spectroscopic imaging (MRSI)

MRSI uses similar principles to conventional MRI scanning to produce spectroscopic analysis based upon the concentrations of endogenous metabolites in the cytosol of the prostatic cells [43]. The levels of citrate produced by normal prostatic epithelial cells are significantly reduced in prostate cancer and this change can be detected in the MRSI spectra.

Recent reports suggest that combined MRI and MRSI scanning may improve upon the ability of conventional MRI to locate prostate cancer and provide staging information [44-46]. Anecdotal reports of the value of MRSI scanning have been published [43] but further studies are required to validate the current findings.

Capromab pendetide

Capromab pendetide (also known as ProstaScint®) is an indium-111 radio-labelled monoclonal antibody to prostate specific membrane antigen. Three to five days following intravenous injection the patient is imaged using planar CT and SPECT [19,47]. Capromab pendetide scanning may be of value in the determination of lymph node status of patients who are due to undergo radical prostatectomy. In one study, the test was found to have a 63% sensitivity, superior in this context to either CT (4%) or MRI (15%). Capromab pendetide scanning gave a 92% negative predictive value for patients with a PSA less than 40ng/ml and a Gleason score less than 7 [48].

Positron emission tomography (PET)

PET depends upon the fact that certain radioisotopes release positrons as they decay, and that these particles can be detected by a nuclear detector and then depicted by CT [49]. Many types of tumours have increased levels of glycolysis compared to normal tissues. The radio-labelled glucose analogue, 18-fluoro-d-glucose (FDG) is commonly used as the tracer in PET. FDG remains trapped in hypermetabolic tumour cells because, unlike glucose-6-phosphate, it is not broken down by glycolysis. This increased activity is what is used to provide the PET images.

FDG-PET has proved of limited use for the detection of localised prostate cancer because of the low metabolic rate of most prostate cancer cells. Both lymph node metastasis and distant metastasis can be identified using FDG-PET and some studies have shown sensitivities and specificity for detection of lymph node metastasis of up to 50%, and 90% respectively [50,51].

Is radiological imaging worthwhile in patients
with clinically localised prostate cancer?

Recommendations	Evidence level

♦ Digital rectal examination may significantly understage or overstage prostate cancer. — IIa/B

♦ TRUS is no better at detecting local extension of prostate cancer than DRE. — III/B

♦ The resolution of CT is too low to be able to distinguish abnormalities within the prostate gland, the state of the capsule, or the presence or absence of disease outside of the prostate gland. — III/B

♦ MRI appears overall to be of limited value in clinically localised prostate cancer, whether palpable or not. However, endorectal MRI can predict extracapsular penetration or seminal vesicle involvement with an accuracy of 84% in patients with clinically localised prostate cancer, a PSA of 10-20ng/ml and a Gleason score of 7 or less. — III/B

♦ MRI is not useful in detecting pelvic node metastasis prior to surgery. — III/B

♦ Isotope bone scans can be avoided in men with clinically localised prostate cancer and a PSA less then 10ng/ml, as the rate of positive scans is very small. — III/B

♦ Newer developments such as SPECT, MRSI, Capromab pendetide, and PET remain largely experimental. Little data are available on the use of SPECT, MRSI and PET in patients with clinically localised prostate cancer. — III/B

♦ Capromab pendetide has shown potential for use in lymph node detection. — III/B

References

1. Clements R, Griffiths GJ, Peeling WB. Staging prostatic cancer. *Clin Radiol* 1992; 46: 225-231.

2. Chodak GW, Keller P, Schoenberg HW. Assessment of screening for prostate cancer using the digital rectal examination. *J Urol* 1989; 141: 1136-1138.

3. Salo JO, Kivisaari L, Rannikko S, Lehtonen T. Computerised tomography and transrectal ultrasound in the assessment of local extension of prostatic cancer before radical retropubic prostatectomy. *J Urol* 1987; 137: 435-438.

4. Ebert T, Schimtz-Dräger BJ, Bürrig K-F, Miller S, Pauli N, Kahn T, Ackermann R. Accuracy of imaging modalities in staging the local extent of prostate cancer. *Urol Clin North Am* 1991; 18: 453-457.

5. Angulo JC, Montie JE, Bukowski T, *et al*. Interobserver consistency of digital rectal examination in clinical staging of localised prostate cancer. *J Urol* 1994; 151: 414A.

6. Narayan P, Gajendran V, Taylor SP, *et al*. The role of transrectal ultrasound-guided biopsy-based staging, preoperative serum prostate-specific antigen and biopsy Gleason score of final pathologic diagnosis in prostate cancer. *Urology* 1995; 46: 205-212.

7. Crawford ED, DeAntoni EP. PSA as a screening test for prostate cancer. *Urol Clin North Am* 1993; 20: (4)637-646.

8. Griffiths GJ, Clements R, Jones DJ, Roberts EE, Peeling WB, Evans KT. The ultrasound appearances of prostatic cancer with histological correlation. *Clin Radiol* 1987; 38: 219-227.

9. Dahnert WF, Hamper UM, Eggleston JC, Walsh PC, Sanders RC. Prostatic evaluation by transrectal sonography with histological correlation: the echopenic appearance of early carcinoma. *Radiology* 1986; 158: 97-102.

10. Schimtz-Dräger BJ, Ebert T, Ackermann R. Clinical staging in carcinoma of the prostate: current aspects. *Recent Results Cancer Res* 1993; 126: 31-42.

11. Rifkin MD, Zerhouni EA, Gatsonis CA, Quint LE, Paushter DM, Epstein JI, Hamper U, Walsh PC, McNeil BJ. Comparison of magnetic resonance imaging and ultrasonography in staging early prostate cancer. Results of a multi-institutional cooperative trial. *N Engl J Med* 1990; 323: 621-6.

12. Maio A, Rifkin MD. Magnetic Resonance imaging of prostate cancer: update. *Topics in Magnetic Resonance Imaging* 1995; 7: (1)54-68.

13. Hricak H, Doms GC, Jeffrey RB, *et al*. Prostate carcinoma: staging by clinical assessment, CT, and MRI. *Radiology* 1987;162:331-336.

14. Galimbu M, Morales P, Al-Askari SA, *et al*. CAT scanning in staging of prostatic cancer. *Urology* 1981; 18: 305-8.

15. Platt JR, Bree RL, Schwab RE. The accuracy of CT in the staging of prostatic carcinoma. *Am J Roentgenol* 1987; 149: 315-318.

16. Cordes M, Tunn UW, Neidl K, Haasner E. Prostatic cancer. Staging via transrectal prostatic sonography and computed tomography with histopathological correlation. *Fortschr Geb Rontgenstr Nuklearmed* 1987; 146(4): 412-4. German.

Is radiological imaging worthwhile in patients
with clinically localised prostate cancer?

Chapter 14

17. Reckwitz T, Potter SR, Partin AW. Prediction of locoregional extension and metastatic disease in prostate cancer: a review. *World J Urol* 2000; 18:165-172.

18. Kattan MW, Eastham JA, Stapleton AM, Wheeler TM, Scardino PT. A preoperative nomogram for disease recurrence following radical prostatectomy for prostate cancer. *J Natl Cancer Inst* 1998; 90(10): 766-771.

19. Moul JW, Kane CJ, Malkowicz SB. The role of imaging studies and molecular markers for selecting candidates for radical prostatectomy. *Urol Clin North Am* 2001; 28(3): 459-472.

20. Bartolozzi C, Crocetti L, Menchi I, Ortori S, Lencioni R. Endorectal magnetic resonance imaging in local staging of prostate carcinoma. *Abdominal Imaging* 2001; 26: 111-122.

21. Schiebler ML, Schnall MD. Pollack HM, *et al*. Current role of MR imaging in the staging of adenocarcinoma of the prostate. *Radiology* 1993; 189: 339-352.

22. Rørvik J, Haukaas S. Magnetic Resonance Imaging of the prostate. *Curr Opin Urol* 2001; 11: 181-188.

23. Vivek D. MR Imaging of the Prostate and seminal vesicles. *MRI Clin North Am* 1996; 4(3): 497-517.

24. Cheng D, Tempany CMC. MR imaging of the prostate and bladder. *Seminars in Ultrasound, CT, and MRI* 1998; 19(1): 67-89.

25. Imaging in the Diagnosis and assessment of prognosis in localized prostate cancer. *Scand J Urol Nephrol* 1994; Suppl 162: 89-106.

26. Adusumilli S, Pretorius ES. Magnetic resonance imaging of prostate cancer. *Sem Urol Oncol* 2002; 20(3): 192-210.

27. Sigelman ES. Magnetic resonance imaging of the prostate. *Seminars in Roentgenology* 1999; 34(4): 295-312.

28. Werner-Wasik M, Whittington R, Malkowicz SB, *et al*. Prostate imaging may not be necessary in nonpalpable carcinoma of the prostate. *Urology* 1997; 50(3): 385-389.

29. D'Amico AV, Whittington R, Malkowicz B, *et al*. Endorectal magnetic resonance imaging as a predictor of biochemical outcome after radical prostatectomy in men with clinically localized prostate cancer. *J Urol* 2000; 164(3 part 1): 759-763.

30. D'Amico AV, Whittington R, Malkowicz SB, *et al*. Critical analysis of the ability of the endorectal coil magnetic resonance imaging scan to predict pathologic stage, margin status, and postoperative prostate-specific antigen failure in patients with clinically organ-confined prostate cancer. *J Clin Oncol* 1996; 14(6): 1770-1777.

31. D'Amico AB, Schnall M, Whittington R, *et al*. Endorectal coil magnetic resonance imaging identifies locally advanced prostate cancer in select patients with clinically localised disease. *J Urol* 1998; 51(3):449-454

32. Ekman P. Predicting pelvic lymph node involvement in patients with localized prostate cancer. *Eur Urol* 1997; 32(suppl 3): 60-64.

33. Pollack HM, Schnall MD. Magnetic resonance imaging in carcinoma of the prostate. The prostate 1992; Suppl 4:17-31

34. David V. MR imaging of the prostate and seminal vesicles. *MRI Clin North Am* 1996; 4: 497-518.

35. Schimtz-Dräger BJ, Ebert T, Ackermann R. Clinical staging in carcinoma of the prostate: current aspects. *Recent Results Cancer Res* 1993; 126: 31-42.

36. Jager GJ, Severens JL, Thornbury JR, *et al*. Prostate cancer staging: Should MR imaging be used? A decision analytic approach. *Radiology* 2000; 215: 445-451.

37. Wolf JS, Cher M, Dall'Era M, *et al*. The use and accuracy of cross-sectional imaging and fine needle aspiration cytology for detection of pelvic lymph node metastases before radical prostatectomy. *J Urol* 1995; 153: 993-999.

38. Engelbrecht MR, Jager GJ, Laheij RJ, *et al*. Local staging of prostate cancer using magnetic resonance imaging: a meta-analysis. *Eur Radiol* 2002; 12: 2294-2302.

39. Alazraki NP, Mishkin FS. Cancer. Alazraki NP, Mishkin FS, Eds. Fundamentals of Nuclear Medicine. Society of Nuclear Medicine, New York, 1984.

40. Chybowski FM, Keller JJ, Bergstralh EJ, *et al*. Predicting radionuclide bone scan findings in patients with newly diagnosed, untreated prostate cancer: prostate specific antigen is superior to all other clinical parameters. *J Urol* 1991; 145: 313-318.

41. Oesterling JE, Martin SK, Bergstralh EJ, *et al*. The use of prostate specific antigen in staging patients with newly diagnosed prostate cancer. *JAMA* 1993; 269: 57-60.

42. Larson SM, Schwartz LH. Advances in imaging. *Sem Oncol* 1994; 21(5): 598-606.

43. Kurhanewicz J, Swanson MG. Nelson SJ, Vigneron DB. Combined magnetic resonance imaging and spectroscopic imaging approach to molecular imaging of prostate cancer. *Journal of Magnetic Resonance Imaging* 2002; 16: 451-463.

44. Scheidler J, Hricak H, Vigneron DB, *et al*. Prostate cancer: localization with three-dimensional proton MR spectroscopic imaging - clinicopathological study. *Radiology* 1999; 213: 473-480.

45. Seltzer SE, Getty DJ, Tempany CMC, *et al*. Staging of Prostate cancer with MR imaging: a combined radiologist-computer system. *Radiology* 1997; 202: 219-226.

46. Yu KK, Scheidler J, Hricak H, *et al*. Improved prediction of extracapsular extension in patients with prostate cancer by the addition of 3D H1-MR spectroscopic imaging to MR imaging. *Radiology* 1999; 213: 481-488.

47. Haseman MK, Rosenthal SA, Polascik TJ. Capromab pendetide imaging of prostate cancer. *Cancer Biotherapy and Radiopharmaceuticals* 2000; 15(2): 131-139.

48. Manyak, MJ, Javitt MC. The role of computerised tomography, magnetic resonance imaging, bone scan, and monoclonal antibody nuclear scan for prognosis prediction in prostate cancer. *Sem Urol Oncol* 1998;16(3):145-152.

49. Shvarts O, Han K, Seltzer M, *et al*. Positron emission tomography in Urologic Oncology. *Cancer Control* 2002; 9(4): 335-341.

50. Kotzerke J, Prang J, Neumaier B, *et al*. Experience with carbon-11 choline positron emission tomography in prostate carcinoma. *Eur J Nucl Med* 2000; 27: 1415-1419.

51. Sanz G, Robles JE, Gimenez M, *et al*. Positron emission tomography with 18fluorine-labeled deoxyglucose: utility in localized and advanced prostate cancer. *Br J Urol* 1999; 84: 1028-1031.

Is radiological imaging worthwhile in patients
with clinically localised prostate cancer?

Chapter 15

Cryoablation or salvage prostatectomy after radiotherapy failure

Fernando Gómez Sancha MD

Consultant Urologist

Instituto de Cirugía Urológica Avanzada, Madrid, Spain

Introduction

Radiation therapy is a main form of treatment for patients with newly diagnosed localised prostate cancer. Twenty-nine percent of men with prostate cancer were treated with radiation therapy in 1996 in USA [1]. Despite refinements in the delivery of radiation to the prostate gland such as intensity modulation, three-dimensional (3D) conformal radiotherapy and computer-guided brachytherapy, approximately 30% of patients will experience a rise in PSA values after radiation-based treatment [2] **(II/B)**. Compared to primary prostate cancer, persistent prostate cancer after radiation therapy represents a more aggressive disease state that kills at least 27% of patients within five years of the first PSA rise [3]. Following radiation therapy 30.6% of pre-treatment diploid tumours were found to be aneuploid after treatment. Similarly, there is a 24% increase in the number of poorly differentiated (Gleason score 8 to 10) tumours after radiotherapy when compared to pre-treatment tumours [3]. Clinical recurrence, either detected by PSA determination or on clinical grounds, predicts ultimate disease dissemination [4,5], shortens disease-specific survival and assigns the subject with a four-fold increase in risk of developing metastatic disease. Many patients will therefore suffer systemic disease and will be incurable when the recurrence is detected, but some will be candidates for potentially curative treatments.

The goal of salvage treatment is to attempt to improve local control and possibly impact long-term survival, but the therapeutic options are somewhat limited. Salvage radical prostatectomy or cysto-prostatectomy are technically difficult procedures that have been associated with high morbidity and prolonged hospital stay. Additional radiation therapy has been tried but still has to prove to be an acceptable treatment option, as these tumours have shown radio-resistance and further radiation may increase the risk of complications [6,7]. Salvage cryosurgery has emerged as a valid and promising alternative for some patients with reduced morbidity [8]. Other options such as photodynamic therapy, are still embryonic [9].

Risk factors for failure after radiation therapy

Patients electing radiation therapy need to be followed indefinitely to detect treatment failure.

Chapter 15

Radiotherapy is not always able to eradicate the cancer due to the relative radio-resistance of prostate cancer (a higher Gleason grade seems to confer higher radio-resistance) and failure to deliver the cytotoxic dose to the whole gland. It is unclear whether the biologic aggressiveness of radio-recurrent prostate cancer is due to time-dependent cancer clonal evolution (potentially induced by radiation damage), or is due to an innately aggressive tumour secondary to over expression or mutation of apoptotic inhibitors that render these tumours resistant to radiation [10]. As prostate cancer is being detected and treated earlier, men nowadays are at risk of progression for a longer time.

Pre-treatment prognostic factors

PSA, stage and grade

The three major pre-treatment prognostic indicators, namely clinical stage, Gleason score and serum PSA level have been found to be associated with disease relapse. PSA, as opposed to clinical stage, determined by digital rectal exam, and to Gleason grading (assigned subjectively by an individual), is a non-subjective test, and remains predictive when subjected to multivariate analysis [11-13] **(II/B)**.

1992 AJCC clinical stage, serum PSA level and Gleason score have been combined to define three risk categories [14] **(IV/C)** as follows:

◆ Low risk (>85% biochemical no evidence of disease [bNED] at five years): T1c-T2a, PSA ≤10ng/mL, Gleason grade ≤6.
◆ Intermediate risk (50% bNED at five years): T2b, PSA 10-20ng/mL, Gleason grade 7.
◆ High risk (33% bNED at five years): T2c or higher, PSA >20ng/mL or Gleason grade >8.

Percentage of positive prostate biopsies

The percentage of positive prostate biopsies ([number of positive cores/number of cores sampled] x 100) has been shown to be an independent predictor of time to postoperative PSA failure [15] **(III/B)**; therefore, this percentage should be considered in conjunction with PSA level, Gleason grade and clinical stage when counselling patients.

Other markers

Other markers, such as expression of tumour suppressor genes and DNA ploidy are under study [16].

Post-treatment prognostic factors

PSA nadir, time to nadir and PSA doubling time

Defining what is the "normal" or desirable PSA after radiotherapy is problematic. After treatment, the prostate experiences glandular atrophy and a reduction in size and number of non-malignant acini that is dose-dependent [17]. Serum PSA declines slowly after radiotherapy because radiation causes post-mitotic cell death, and fatally damaged cells may survive and divide a limited number of times before apoptosis takes place [18]. Absolute PSA nadir, time to nadir and PSA doubling time have been correlated to the radiation failure pattern [19,20] **(III/B)**. There are three potential sources of PSA after radiotherapy: residual benign epithelium (no evidence of disease), residual cancer cells (local failure) and subclinical micrometastases (distant failure). The longer the time to nadir and the lower the nadir value, the more likely it is that treatment has been successful and that there are no micrometastases or residual prostatic cancer cells. When there are active residual cancer cells in the prostate, PSA declines progressively until the growth rate of these cancer cells is greater than the death rate of those damaged by radiation, and it is then that PSA starts to rise. If there were micrometastases undetected prior to treatment, these are not affected by local treatment, and thus, an earlier and higher nadir will take place. The combination of PSA nadir, time to nadir and PSA doubling time help to determine the failure pattern in the individual patient (Table 1). Neoadjuvant androgen deprivation is often used with radiotherapy, especially in high risk patients; this makes the interpretation of PSA as an indicator of radiation response more difficult.

Table 1. Failure pattern according to level of PSA nadir, time to nadir and PSA doubling time. Modified from [14].

Pattern	No evidence of disease	Local failure	Distant failure
PSA nadir	0.4-0.5 ng/mL	2-3 ng/mL	5-10 ng/mL
Time to nadir	22-23 months	10-12 months	17-20 months
PSA doubling time	NA	11-13 months	3-6 months

Post-radiotherapy biopsy

The difficulty of interpreting the histology of post-radiation prostate specimens has motivated the adoption of PSA as a surrogate endpoint to determine treatment efficacy. Biopsies performed soon after radiotherapy show moderate to marked radiation effect and pathologists are unable to predict viability of these cells. Apparently, the optimal timing for prostate biopsies is 30-36 months post-radiation, as in one study, 30% of positive prostate biopsies at 12-18 months subsequently cleared 12 to 18 months later after treatment [21]. Biopsies are performed under TRUS guidance, and a false-negative rate of 19% (demonstrated by a second positive set of biopsies) has been reported. Prostate biopsies are useful for distinguishing between local and distant failure and are indicated prior to considering salvage treatment.

Diagnosis of recurrence

Digital rectal examination (DRE)

DRE has a specificity of 57% and sensitivity of 41% based on biopsy results, and it has been suggested that it can be omitted from follow-up protocols [22], due to the fact that all suspicious lesions were detected in the context of PSA rises. Between 20%-80% of patients with positive post-radiation biopsies may have a normal DRE [23,24] (III/B).

PSA monitoring

There has been a lack of consensus in the definition of biochemical failure that has complicated

the understanding of radio-resistant prostate cancer behaviour and response to treatment, as different investigators have used different PSA thresholds to define biochemical failure. The 1996 ASTRO Consensus Conference [25] (IV/C) defined biochemical recurrence as three consecutive serum PSA rises in determinations performed at 3-4 month intervals during the first two years after radiotherapy and every six months thereafter. The contribution of this consensus is the concept that there is no distinct PSA threshold that defines successful treatment, and that it is more important to consider PSA stability after reaching the nadir value. This definition is used for the purposes of clinical trials and the reporting of data, and establishes the date of failure to the midterm between the PSA nadir and the date of the first increase. It is important to stress the fact that establishing that a patient meets the criteria for biochemical recurrence does not always justify intervention.

Prostate biopsy

If a patient is suspected of having persistent prostate cancer due to a change on DRE, clinical signs or symptoms of systemic disease or a rising PSA, he should undergo an ultrasound-guided prostate needle biopsy, including cores from the seminal vesicles.

Metastatic work-up

When salvage therapy is being considered, a metastatic work-up is mandatory. This must include computed tomography or magnetic resonance imaging of the abdomen and pelvis, chest radiographs and bone scan. Whereas it is unusual in the pre-treatment setting to have metastatic disease in the absence of PSA greater than 10ng/mL, it is important to remember that this cut-off does not apply in post-radiation patients. Clinical understaging of these radio-resistant malignancies is common and only approximately 20%-40% of these tumours are actually organ-confined on final pathologic examination. There may be a role in performing an open or laparoscopic lymph node dissection of the pelvic lymph nodes (20%-40% of patients in the salvage prostatectomy series have positive nodes), which can be technically challenging, or in performing a ProstaScint® scan, although this still remains controversial.

Treatment options

It is difficult to compare and contrast both main salvage options: salvage cryosurgery and salvage radical prostatectomy because of:

◆ the retrospective, single institution nature of most studies;
◆ the non-uniform patient selection; and
◆ the variations in the definition of biochemical failure [26].

Salvage radical prostatectomy

Radical prostatectomy has been successful in eradicating locally recurrent cancer after definitive radiotherapy, but with a high complication rate [27-32].

Patient selection

Patient selection is of utmost importance. Quality of life, co-existent medical conditions and longevity should be assessed and balanced with the morbidity of this surgical procedure. It is usually reserved for patients in excellent health with a life expectancy of at least ten years who had clinically localised disease prior to the initial radiation treatment, a biopsy-proven recurrence >18 months after primary treatment and a negative metastatic work-up. This operation is only for highly motivated patients who are aware of the high

rate of complications. Candidates should be treated before the PSA level rises above 10ng/mL, as pre-operative serum PSA levels have a positive correlation with pathologic stage. If the pre-operative PSA level was less than 10ng/mL, only 15% of patients have advanced pathologic features, compared with 86% if the PSA level was higher than 10ng/mL.

Technique

Patients are prepared for surgery with a thorough mechanical and antibiotic bowel preparation. They must be aware that if the procedure is not feasible, based on intra-operative findings, a cysto-prostatectomy might be obligatory, and that it could be aborted if frozen sections show metastatic disease. Salvage prostatectomy can be approached in either a retropubic [33], perineal [34] or laparoscopic [35] fashion **(III/B)**. The perineal approach does not allow sampling of the pelvic nodes. The surgeon choosing a retropubic route must be ready to modify his approach as the intra-operative situation dictates, choosing an antegrade vs. retrograde dissection or a retroperitoneal vs. an intraperitoneal approach [27]. Several indications for cystoprostatectomy have been described [36]: biopsy-confirmed bladder neck or seminal vesicle invasion, incontinence as a result of a non-compliant, irradiated bladder, and any intractable manifestations of radiation cystitis. Results of cystoprostatectomy are poor, as in two studies only 10%-16% of patients exhibited organ-confined disease [30,33]; cystoprostatectomy does not benefit the patient with an advanced stage of local recurrence.

Efficacy

Rates of recurrence and disease-free survival following salvage surgery for locally recurrent prostate cancer are strongly predicted by the final pathologic stage [27,30]. The actuarial non-progression rate at five years was 57% and at ten years, 35%. The five-year actuarial non-progression rate was 100% for patients with organ-confined cancer, 71% for those with extracapsular extension, and 28% for those with seminal vesicle invasion. Stage for stage, results are comparable to those of standard radical prostatectomy [27] **(III/B)**.

Morbidity

Salvage surgery is associated with significantly greater morbidity than standard radical prostatectomy. The most commonly reported complications include rectal injury (0%-19%) (Figure 1), urinary incontinence (0%-64%) (Figure 2), bladder neck contracture (17%-25%), and lymphoedema (10%) [37] **(III/B)**. Erectile dysfunction is almost inevitable, although sural nerve grafts have been used in pre-operatively potent patients. Furthermore, as many as 25% of patients will experience other complications such as prolonged urinary extravasation, deep venous thrombosis, wound infection or pulmonary embolism.

Salvage cryosurgery

Cryosurgery has been utilised for the treatment of a wide variety of diseases, including skin, liver, prostate and kidney tumours. It relies on the fact that very cold temperatures delivered in a rapid fashion can result in lethal injury to individual cells. Cryobiological experiments identified the basic features of the optimal cryosurgical approach; a rapid freezing followed by a slow thaw process repeated over a number of cycles (freeze-thaw cycles), that results in irreversible cellular damage through several mechanisms.

Prostate cryosurgery has undergone several phases of development; the initial technique involved

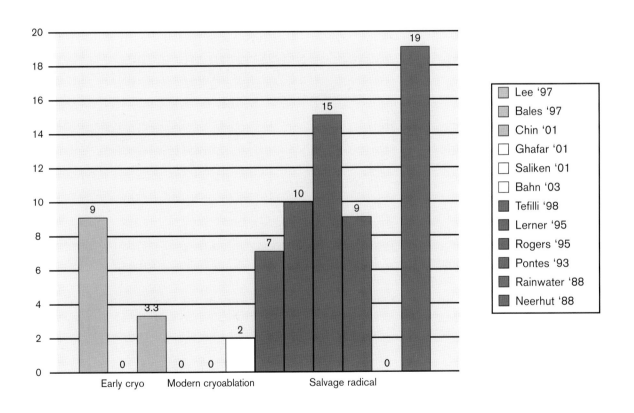

Figure 1. Rectal injury following salvage cryosurgery and salvage radical prostatectomy. Modern cryoablation technical enhancements have led to a reduction of rectal injury [8,27,33,39,43,44,47,52-54,56,57].

Chapter 15

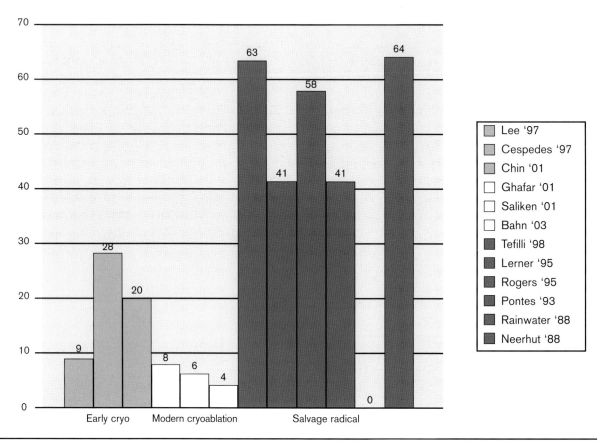

Figure 2. Incontinence following salvage cryosurgery and salvage radical prostatectomy. Enhancements in cryosurgical technique (urethral warming and temperature monitoring at the sphincter level) have led to an improvement in the incontinence rate after cryosurgery [8,27,31,33,39,43,47,51-55].

an open perineal incision with placement of probes under direct visual and digital control, and relied on liquid nitrogen pumped through the probes to generate cold temperatures. The high complication rate of this approach, due to injury of adjacent organs, made the procedure unpopular among urologists. Onik *et al* [38] described a transperineal technique for prostate cancer cryoablation with transrectal ultrasound monitoring of the procedure, which allowed for better control of the propagation of the ice ball preventing damage to surrounding structures. Recent advances in technology and standardisation of the surgical methodology have led to more widespread application of the procedure, with corresponding improvements in efficacy and safety [39].

These advances are:

♦ The use of argon gas to induce freezing instead of liquid nitrogen, with the additional advantage of using helium gas to thaw, which allows for a better control of the freeze-thaw cycle.
♦ The use of thermocouple devices that measure real time temperatures in critical anatomical landmarks (neurovascular bundles, Denonvilliers, prostatic apex, external sphincter).
♦ The use of an FDA approved urethral warming device, that prevents postoperative tissue sloughing.
♦ The use of two or more freeze-thaw cycles and six or more cryoprobes [40].

- The use of computer-guided systems that provide intra-operative treatment planning, with a potential for increased tissue destruction [41]. It is therefore very important to identify the methodology used for cryoablation of the prostate when interpreting published results.

Modern prostate cryosurgery is considered a reasonable option for primary localised and locally advanced prostate cancer treatment in selected patients [42]. The high rate of complications of salvage radical prostatectomy led to the investigation of the potential utility of this approach for radio-resistant prostate cancer.

Patient selection

Currently, there are no defined guidelines to select patients properly for salvage cryoablation. The optimal candidates would be those patients that are candidates for localised therapy. Patients with a previous history of transurethral resection of the prostate (TURP), invasion of seminal vesicles or lymph nodes should be excluded from cryosurgery. Bahn's et al seven-year follow-up retrospective study on salvage cryoablation suggests that a favourable outcome can be expected if cryoablation is performed when post-radiation serum PSA is <10ng/mL and tumour stage is T1-T2 [8] **(III/B)**.

Technique

Patients are given an enema on the morning of the procedure and prophylactic antibiotics. The procedure is performed under spinal anaesthesia. A suprapubic catheter is placed under cystoscopic guidance, and the bladder is left distended; alternatively, a Foley catheter is left after the procedure. A urethral warming catheter is inserted prior to freezing the tissue and is maintained at 38°C to 42°C for two hours postoperatively. Six to eight cryoprobes are positioned under TRUS guidance, and thermocouple devices are placed adjacent to both neurovascular bundles, prostatic apex, Denonvillier's fascia and external sphincter. Freezing is performed activating sequentially anterior probes and then posterior probes until all prostatic tissue appears to be frozen on TRUS, and thermocouple readings at neurovascular bundles show temperatures under - 40°C. The thermocouples at the external sphincter, apex and Denonvillier's fascia allow control of the safety of the freezing process. If the temperature at the sphincter reaches 0°C, the freezing is stopped and thawing starts; this seems to prevent postoperative incontinence. When temperatures are satisfactory, the argon gas is stopped, and helium gas starts to circulate through the probes; this thaws the prostate and prevents further ice ball expansion. At least two freeze-thaw cycles are used. Some groups advocate injecting saline in the Denonvillier's space, to allow for a safer freezing of the peripheral zone of the prostate, as well as injecting warm saline in the rectum as an additional precaution. Most patients are discharged within 24 hours.

Efficacy

Figure 3 shows the range of biochemical disease-free survival (BDFS) rates published with a five-year follow-up after salvage cryoablation and salvage prostatectomy. Results from salvage cryosurgery series are summarised in Table 2. It is remarkable in the study from Chin et al [43] that the overall negative biopsy rate was 97%; this included biopsy data from over 700 cores of tissue with a median follow-up of 18.6 months. It is also interesting that in those patients with positive biopsies after cryosurgery, these became negative after a second cryoablation. The seven-year BDFS data from the report from Bahn et al [8] further supports cryoablation as a safe and efficacious salvage treatment option for radio-resistant prostate cancer with durable results **(III/B)**.

Morbidity

Over the past decade, several institutions have published their salvage cryosurgery results. Early series reported a significant number of complications [44], but these have diminished in recent series using state-of-the-art cryosurgical techniques. Complications are more frequent after salvage cryoablation when compared to cryoablation as a primary treatment. The major complications described after salvage cryoablation with argon-based systems are rectal

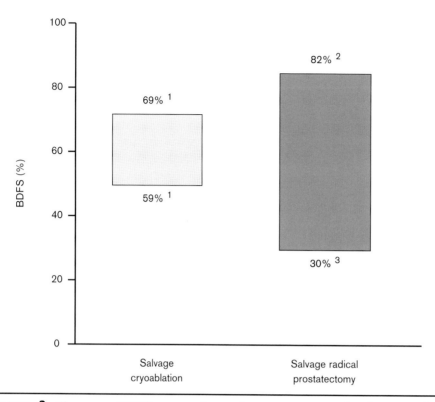

Figure 3. Five-year BDFS comparison of cryosurgery and salvage radical prostatectomy. Range of published results. 1=Bahn *et al* [8], 2=Zincke *et al* [49], 3=Brenner *et al* [50].

Table 2. Results of salvage cryosurgery studies.

Study	N	Follow-up (months)	BRFS / local control rate	Positive prostate biopsy
Pisters (1997) [46]	150 total	13.5 (1.2-32.2)	-	25/100 (23%) patients
	71 single freeze	17.3	37% BRFS§	29% patients
	79 double freeze	10	66% BRFS§	7% patients
Lee (1997) [47]	43	-	65% local control rate	At 3 months 3/20 (15%) patients
				At 1 year 7/20 (35%) patients
Miller (1996) [48]	33	17.1 (4.1-34.3)	-	9/33 (27.3%) patients
Chin (2001) [43]	118 patients 125 procedures	18.6 (3-54)	68% BRFS*	23/745 (3%) cores 7 patients
Katz (2003) [45]	43	21.9 (1.2-54)	7 months: 79% BRFS 12 months: 66% BRFS	3/8 (37%) patients
Bahn (2003) [8]	59	72.5	59%* BRFS 69%† BRFS	0/38 (0%) patients

BRFS=biochemical recurrence-free survival (Kaplan-Meier curve analysis); * With a PSA cut-off of 0.5ng/mL; † With a PSA cut-off of 1ng/mL; § Biochemical failure defined as an increase in serum PSA of 0.2ng/mL above the nadir value.

injury (0%-3%), incontinence (4%-8%), impotence (72%) and urethral sloughing or obstruction requiring transurethral resection of the prostate (0%-4%). Minor complications were perineal pain or rectal discomfort (26%), transient perineal or scrotal oedema (12%), lower urinary tract infection (9%) and mild haematuria (5%) [45] **(III/B)**.

Conclusions

Radio-resistant prostate cancer is a serious health risk for approximately 30% of patients treated with primary radiation therapy for localised prostate cancer. Most patients carry large volume and poorly differentiated disease at the time of diagnosis, which limits the ability of salvage therapy to eradicate the cancer. The goal of disease eradication must be balanced against the potential for serious treatment-related side effects. Salvage radical prostatectomy achieves good results when radio-resistant cancer is confined to the prostate gland, but with a high morbidity. The main problem lies in the difficulty of selecting the right patient for such an aggressive approach. Salvage cryoablation is a promising less invasive treatment option with reduced morbidity and no known latent complications, that has shown to be able to eradicate cancer from the prostate gland. Other options such as salvage brachytherapy and photodynamic therapy are still investigational.

Acknowledgement

I would like to thank Dr. John Rewcastle for his assistance and comments in the preparation of the tables. Conflicts of interest: None.

Chapter 15

Chapter 15

Recommendations	Evidence level

How frequent is radiation-resistant prostate cancer?

- Approximately 30% of patients will experience a PSA rise after radiation-based treatment. — II/B

What are the risk factors for failure after radiation therapy?

- Pre-treatment prognostic factors are: the combination of PSA, Gleason score and clinical stage, which allow stratification of patients into low, medium and high risk groups. The percentage of positive prostate biopsies must also be taken into account. — III/B
- Post-treatment prognostic factors are: PSA nadir, time to nadir and PSA doubling time. Prostate biopsy 30-36 months after radiation. — III/B

How is a recurrence diagnosed?

- DRE could be omitted from follow-up protocols. — III/B
- Three consecutive PSA rises after nadir (ASTRO definition). — IV/C
- Prostate biopsy including cores from seminal vesicles.
- Metastatic work-up even with a low PSA.

Comparison of treatment options

- This is difficult to compare and contrast, due to the retrospective nature of most studies, the non-uniform patient selection and the variations in the definition of biochemical failure used.

Salvage radical prostatectomy/cystoprostatectomy

- Patient selection is important: young, biopsy-proven recurrence, a PSA <10ng/mL, awareness of complications.
- Retropubic, perineal and laparoscopic approaches are feasible. — III/B
- The efficacy is comparable stage by stage to standard radical prostatectomy. Five-year BDFS ranges from 30% to 82%. — III/B
- High morbidity. — III/B

Salvage cryosurgery

- Patients with T1-T2 disease, PSA <10ng/mL. It is not feasible in patients who have had a previous TURP, invasion of seminal vesicles. — III/B
- It is able to eradicate cancer from the gland (negative biopsy rate 97%). Five-year BDFS ranges from 59% to 69%. — III/B
- Lower morbidity. — III/B

References

1. Mettlin CJ, Murphy GP, McDonald CJ, Menck HR. The National Cancer Data base report on increased use of brachytherapy for the treatment of patients with prostate carcinoma in the U.S. *Cancer* 1999; 86(9): 1877-1882.
2. Brawer MK. Radiation therapy failure in prostate cancer patients: risk factors and methods of detection. *Rev Urol* 2002; 4((Suppl 2): S1): 2-11.
3. Siders DB, Lee F. Histologic changes of irradiated prostatic carcinoma diagnosed by transrectal ultrasound. *Hum Pathol* 1992; 23(4): 344-351.
4. Fuks Z, Leibel SA, Wallner KE, Begg CB, Fair WR, Anderson LL, *et al*. The effect of local control on metastatic dissemination in carcinoma of the prostate: long-term results in patients treated with 125I implantation. *Int J Radiat Oncol Biol Phys* 1991; 21(3): 537-547.
5. Kaplan ID, Prestidge BR, Bagshaw MA, Cox RS. The importance of local control in the treatment of prostatic cancer. *J Urol* 1992; 147(3 Pt 2): 917-921.
6. Beyer DC. Brachytherapy for recurrent prostate cancer after radiation therapy. *Semin Radiat Oncol* 2003; 13(2): 158-165.
7. Grado GL, Collins JM, Kriegshauser JS, Balch CS, Grado MM, Swanson GP, *et al*. Salvage brachytherapy for localized prostate cancer after radiotherapy failure. *Urology* 1999; 53(1): 2-10.
8. Bahn DK, Lee F, Silverman P, Bahn J, Badalament R, Kumar A, *et al*. Salvage cryosurgery for recurrent prostate cancer after radiation therapy: a 7-year follow-up. *Clinical Prostate Cancer*. In Press, 2003.
9. Nathan TR, Whitelaw DE, Chang SC, Lees WR, Ripley PM, Payne H, *et al*. Photodynamic therapy for prostate cancer recurrence after radiotherapy: a phase I study. *J Urol* 2002; 168(4 Pt 1): 1427-1432.
10. Steinberg GD. Salvage radical prostatectomy for radio-recurrent prostate cancer: is this a viable option? *Curr Opin Urol* 2000; 10(3): 229-232.
11. Lee WR, Hanks GE, Schultheiss TE, Corn BW, Hunt MA. Localized prostate cancer treated by external-beam radiotherapy alone: serum prostate-specific antigen-driven outcome analysis. *J Clin Oncol* 1995; 13(2): 464-469.
12. Kupelian PA, Katcher J, Levin H, *et al*. External beam radiotherapy versus radical prostatectomy for clinical stage T1-2 prostate cancer: therapeutic implications of stratification by pretreatment PSA levels and biopsy Gleason Scores. *Cancer J Sci Am* 1997; 3: 78-87.
13. Zagars GK, Pollack A, Kavadi VS, Von Eschenbach AC. Prostate-specific antigen and radiation therapy for clinically localized prostate cancer. *Int J Radiat Oncol Biol Phys* 1995; 32(2): 293-306.
14. D'Amico AV, Crook J, Beard CJ, DeWeese TL, Hurwitz M, Kaplan ID. Radiation therapy for prostate cancer. In: *Campbell's Urology*. Walsh PC, Retik AB, Darracott Vaughan Jr. E, Wein AJ, Kavoussi LR, Novick AC, *et al*, Eds. Saunders, New York, 2002: 3147-3170.
15. D'Amico AV, Whittington R, Malkowicz SB, Schultz D, Silver B, Henry L, *et al*. Clinical utility of percent-positive prostate biopsies in predicting biochemical outcome after radical prostatectomy or external-beam radiation therapy for patients with clinically localized prostate cancer. *Mol Urol* 2000; 4(3): 171-175.
16. Pollack A, Grignon DJ, Heydon KH, Hammond EH, Lawton CA, Mesic JB, *et al*. Prostate cancer DNA ploidy and response to salvage hormone therapy after radiotherapy with or without short-term total androgen blockade: an analysis of RTOG 8610. *J Clin Oncol* 2003; 21(7): 1238-1248.
17. Critz FA, Williams WH, Holladay CT, Levinson AK, Benton JB, Holladay DA, *et al*. Post-treatment PSA < or = 0.2ng/mL defines disease freedom after radiotherapy for prostate cancer using modern techniques. *Urology* 1999; 54(6): 968-971.
18. Mostofi FK, Sesterhenn IA, Davis CJ, Jr. A pathologist's view of prostatic carcinoma. *Cancer* 1993; 71(3 Suppl): 906-932.
19. Lee WR, Hanlon AL, Hanks GE. Prostate specific antigen nadir following external beam radiation therapy for clinically localized prostate cancer: the relationship between nadir level and disease-free survival. *J Urol* 1996; 156(2 Pt 1): 450-453.
20. Kestin LL, Vicini FA, Ziaja EL, Stromberg JS, Frazier RC, Martinez AA. Defining biochemical cure for prostate carcinoma patients treated with external beam radiation therapy. *Cancer* 1999; 86(8): 1557-1566.
21. Crook J, Malone S, Perry G, Bahadur Y, Robertson S, Abdolell M. Postradiotherapy prostate biopsies: what do they really mean? Results for 498 patients. *Int J Radiat Oncol Biol Phys* 2000; 48(2): 355-367.
22. Johnstone PA, McFarland JT, Riffenburgh RH, Amling CL. Efficacy of digital rectal examination after radiotherapy for prostate cancer. *J Urol* 2001; 166(5): 1684-1687.
23. Kabalin JN, Hodge KK, McNeal JE, Freiha FS, Stamey TA. Identification of residual cancer in the prostate following radiation therapy: role of transrectal ultrasound guided biopsy and prostate specific antigen. *J Urol* 1989; 142(2 Pt 1): 326-331.
24. Scardino PT, Frankel JM, Wheeler TM, Meacham RB, Hoffman GS, Seale C, *et al*. The prognostic significance of post-irradiation biopsy results in patients with prostatic cancer. *J Urol* 1986; 135(3): 510-516.
25. Panel AsfTRaOC. Consensus Statement: guidelines for PSA following radiation therapy. *Int J Radiat Oncol Biol Phys* 1997; 37: 1035-1041.
26. Long JP, Bahn D, Lee F, Shinohara K, Chinn DO, Macaluso JN, Jr. Five-year retrospective, multi-institutional pooled analysis of cancer-related outcomes after cryosurgical ablation of the prostate. *Urology* 2001; 57(3): 518-523.
27. Rogers E, Ohori M, Kassabian VS, Wheeler TM, Scardino PT. Salvage radical prostatectomy: outcome measured by serum prostate specific antigen levels. *J Urol* 1995; 153(1): 104-110.
28. Cheng L, Sebo TJ, Slezak J, Pisansky TM, Bergstralh EJ, Neumann RM, *et al*. Predictors of survival for prostate carcinoma patients treated with salvage radical prostatectomy after radiation therapy. *Cancer* 1998; 83(10): 2164-2171.
29. Garzotto M, Wajsman Z. Androgen deprivation with salvage surgery for radiorecurrent prostate cancer: results at 5-year follow-up. *J Urol* 1998; 159(3): 950-954.

30. Gheiler EL, Tefilli MV, Tiguert R, Grignon D, Cher ML, Sakr W, et al. Predictors for maximal outcome in patients undergoing salvage surgery for radio-recurrent prostate cancer. Urology 1998; 51(5): 789-795.

31. Tefilli MV, Gheiler EL, Tiguert R, Banerjee M, Forman J, Pontes JE, et al. Salvage surgery or salvage radiotherapy for locally recurrent prostate cancer. Urology 1998; 52(2): 224-229.

32. Miles BJ, Herman JR, Reiter RE, Scardino PT. Salvage radical prostatectomy for local recurrence of prostate cancer after radiation therapy. In: Comprehensive Textbook of Genitourinary Oncology. Vogelzang NJ, Shipley WU, Scardino PT, Coffey DS, Eds. Lippincott Williams & Wilkins, Philadelphia, 2000: 813-823.

33. Lerner SE, Blute ML, Zincke H. Critical evaluation of salvage surgery for radio-recurrent/resistant prostate cancer. J Urol 1995; 154(3): 1103-1109.

34. Ziada A, Lisle T, Price B. Salvage prostatectomy after radiation therapy: experience using the perineal approach. Grand Rounds Urol 1998; 1(15).

35. Vallancien G, Gupta R, Cathelineau X, Baumert H, Rozet F. Initial results of salvage laparoscopic radical prostatectomy after radiation failure. J Urol 2003; 170(5): 1838-1840.

36. Corral DA, Pisters LL, Von Eschenbach AC. Treatment options for localized recurrence of prostate cancer following radiation therapy. Urol Clin North Am 1996; 23(4): 677-684.

37. Pontes JE. Role of surgery in managing local recurrence following external-beam radiation therapy. Urol Clin North Am 1994; 21(4): 701-706.

38. Onik GM, Cohen JK, Reyes GD, Rubinsky B, Chang Z, Baust J. Transrectal ultrasound-guided percutaneous radical cryosurgical ablation of the prostate. Cancer 1993; 72(4): 1291-1299.

39. Ghafar MA, Johnson CW, De La TA, Benson MC, Bagiella E, Fatal M, et al. Salvage cryotherapy using an argon-based system for locally recurrent prostate cancer after radiation therapy: the Columbia experience. J Urol 2001; 166(4): 1333-1337.

40. Larson TR, Rrobertson DW, Corica A, Bostwick DG. In vivo interstitial temperature mapping of the human prostate during cryosurgery with correlation to histopathologic outcomes. Urology 2000; 55(4): 547-552.

41. Jankun M, Kelly TJ, Zaim A, Young K, Keck RW, Selman SH, et al. Computer model for cryosurgery of the prostate. Comput Aided Surg 1999; 4(4): 193-199.

42. Bahn DK, Lee F, Badalament R, Kumar A, Greski J, Chernick M. Targeted cryoablation of the prostate: 7-year outcomes in the primary treatment of prostate cancer. Urology 2002; 60(2 Suppl 1):3-11.

43. Chin JL, Pautler SE, Mouraviev V, Touma N, Moore K, Downey DB. Results of salvage cryoablation of the prostate after radiation: identifying predictors of treatment failure and complications. J Urol 2001; 165(6 Pt 1): 1937-1941.

44. Bales GT, Williams MJ, Sinner M, Thisted RA, Chodak GW. Short-term outcomes after cryosurgical ablation of the prostate in men with recurrent prostate carcinoma following radiation therapy. Urology 1995; 46(5): 676-680.

45. Katz AE. Salvage cryoablation of the prostate. In: Prostate Cancer Science and Clinical Practice. Mydlo JH, Godec CJ, Eds. Academic Press, New York, 2003: 451-457.

46. Pisters LL, Von Eschenbach AC, Scott SM, Swanson DA, Dinney CP, Pettaway CA, et al. The efficacy and complications of salvage cryotherapy of the prostate. J Urol 1997; 157(3): 921-925.

47. Lee F, Bahn DK, McHugh TA, Kumar AA, Badalament RA. Cryosurgery of prostate cancer. Use of adjuvant hormonal therapy and temperature monitoring - a one year follow-up. Anticancer Res 1997; 17(3A): 1511-1515.

48. Miller RJ, Jr., Cohen JK, Shuman B, Merlotti LA. Percutaneous, transperineal cryosurgery of the prostate as salvage therapy for post radiation recurrence of adenocarcinoma. Cancer 1996; 77(8): 1510-1514.

49. Zincke H. Radical prostatectomy and exenterative procedures for local failure after radiotherapy with curative intent: comparison of outcomes. J Urol 1992; 147(3 Pt 2): 894-899.

50. Brenner PC, Russo P, Wood DP, Morse MJ, Donat SM, Fair WR. Salvage radical prostatectomy in the management of locally recurrent prostate cancer after 125I implantation. Br J Urol 1995; 75(1): 44-47.

51. Cespedes RD, Pisters LL, Von Eschenbach AC, McGuire EJ. Long-term follow-up of incontinence and obstruction after salvage cryosurgical ablation of the prostate: results in 143 patients. J Urol 1997; 157(1): 237-240.

52. Saliken JC, Donnelly BJ, Ernst S, Rewcastle J, Wiseman D. Prostate cryotherapy: practicalities and applications from the Calgary experience. Can Assoc Radiol J 2001; 52(3):165-173.

53. Pontes JE, Montie J, Klein E, Huben R. Salvage surgery for radiation failure in prostate cancer. Cancer 1993; 71(3 Suppl): 976-980.

54. Rainwater LM, Zincke H. Radical prostatectomy after radiation therapy for cancer of the prostate: feasibility and prognosis. J Urol 1988; 140(6): 1455-1459.

55. Neerhut GJ, Wheeler T, Cantini M, Scardino PT. Salvage radical prostatectomy for radiorecurrent adenocarcinoma of the prostate. J Urol 1988; 140(3): 544-549.

56. Tefilli MV, Gheiler EL, Tiguert R, Barroso U, Jr., Barton CD, Wood DP, Jr., et al. Quality of life in patients undergoing salvage procedures for locally recurrent prostate cancer. J Surg Oncol 1998; 69(3): 156-161.

57. Neerhut GJ, Wheeler T, Cantini M, Scardino PT. Salvage radical prostatectomy for radiorecurrent adenocarcinoma of the prostate. J Urol 1988; 140(3): 544-549.

Chapter 16

Localised prostate cancer: a case history-based look at the evidence

Mark R Feneley MD FRCS (Eng) FRCS (Urol), Senior Lecturer in Urological Oncology [1]
Roger Kirby MD FRCS (Urol) FEBU, Professor of Urology [2]
Robert Lee MD, Professor and Vice-Chairman [3]
Alison Birtle MRCP FRCR, Senior Specialist Registrar, Clinical Oncology [4]
Heather Payne MRCP FRCR, Consultant Clinical Oncologist [5]
Chris Parker BA MRCP MD FRCR, Senior Lecturer in Clinical Oncology [6]

1 INSTITUTE OF UROLOGY AND NEPHROLOGY, UNIVERSITY COLLEGE LONDON, LONDON, UK
2 ST GEORGE'S HOSPITAL, LONDON, UK
3 DEPARTMENT OF RADIATION ONCOLOGY, WAKE FOREST UNIVERSITY SCHOOL OF MEDICINE, WINSTON-SALEM, NC, USA
4 THE ROYAL MARSDEN HOSPITAL, SUTTON, SURREY, UK
5 THE MEYERSTEIN INSTITUTE OF ONCOLOGY, THE MIDDLESEX HOSPITAL, LONDON, UK
6 INSTITUTE OF CANCER RESEARCH & THE ROYAL MARSDEN HOSPITAL, SUTTON, SURREY, UK

Introduction

The area of prostate cancer cure is one of great controversy at present, with wild claims and counter-claims being made for various therapeutic options while few good comparative studies have ever been carried out. As van Poppel shows in Chapter 20, the provider of a treatment may influence outcome as much as the treatment chosen.

With this in mind, we decided to ask experts in each of four camps to give an overview of the evidence for and against one treatment, based on a series of case vignettes. Each of these is based on a real patient who presented to one of the editor's practice seeking advice.

The treatments and their protagonists are:

Radical prostatectomy:
Mark Feneley and Roger Kirby
Interstitial brachytherapy:
Robert Lee
External beam radiotherapy:
Alison Birtle and Heather Payne
Active surveillance:
Chris Parker

It will be noted that each of the authors stresses the need to fully involve the patient in treatment decisions in this area, where few if any direct comparative studies exist. Dr Parker felt that for the majority of the cases presented, the case for active surveillance could not be made on current evidence and for this,

Chapter 16

and to Dr Lee, we perhaps owe an editor's apology for choosing cases at the extreme ends of the management conundrum!

Lastly, it is difficult in all cases to assess the level of evidence, since so few RCTs have been carried out or even attempted in these patients. Most of the references quoted are from case series, usually without controls. A question for the future is whether or not we should be attempting to remedy what is seen by many as a deficiency in our management of prostate cancer, namely the relative absence of level I and II evidence. However, the data given by the authors here comes from years of experience from hundreds of institutions and many thousands of patients.

Case 1

A 48-year-old black man with a positive family history (three dead from prostate cancer) is found to have a PSA of 3.6ug/l at screening, with normal DRE. He is potent and has an IPSS of 16 (moderate bother). Biopsies have shown Gleason pattern 3 cancer in two out of ten cores (both on the same side with 30% of each core involved).

Radical prostatectomy: Case 1

This patient has been diagnosed with prostate cancer at an early clinical stage, and he has the opportunity for definitive, potentially curative treatment **(Ib/A)**. Radical prostatectomy is the most definitive treatment for organ-confined prostate cancer [1] and achieves excellent long-term cancer-free survival in men with clinically localised disease [2]. It also provides additional pathological information that may be valuable for prognostic assessment, and thereby may influence subsequent intervention [3]. This man's relatively young age at diagnosis is a favourable factor influencing outcome with radical prostatectomy [4]. However, the natural history of PSA-detected prostate cancer without early definitive intervention and the risk of metastatic progression or prostate cancer death are not well defined, with most long-term studies reporting from the pre-PSA era [5,6]. Epidemiological studies have not shown that younger age is an

adverse prognostic factor; however, a younger individual will be at long-term (lifetime) risk of disease progression without treatment, and the impact of metastatic progression may be more substantial in terms of lost life expectancy.

A black man with a family history of prostate cancer must be considered to be at greater risk of developing and dying from prostate cancer than an age-matched white Caucasian **(IIa/B)**. Some studies suggest that US blacks have more advanced stage disease at diagnosis and worse stage-adjusted survival than whites. Others propose that blacks have a worse phenotype, even adjusted for stage, associated with higher PSA levels and higher Gleason grade [7]. Serum PSA levels may be independently prognostic and differences in exposure to testing may also contribute to outcomes [8]. Disease-related outcomes may also be substantially influenced by racial differences in disease biology, comorbidity, sociocultural and environmental factors, also impacting on treatment opportunities [9,10]. The overall impact of race and family history on outcome following screening and treatment is not defined well, particularly in relation to other established prognostic factors [11,12]. Differences however, may be reduced by the stage shift associated with PSA testing [13], and especially after adjusting for clinical stage, Gleason score and serum PSA [14,15].

The biopsy findings in this patient suggest that his tumour is potentially curable **(Ib/A)**. Two of 10 cores show Gleason 3 in around 30%, indicating a biopsy sum score of 6, represented unilaterally. It is well recognised that tumour grade can be misrepresented in the needle cores, and the more adverse prognosis associated with higher grade may therefore be unrecognised at this time. Partin's tables for prediction of pathological stage take into consideration other independent pre-operative variables including clinical stage and serum PSA [16], and indicate a good probability of favourable pathology, including organ-confined disease **(IIa/B)**. There have been a growing number of other nomograms published in recent years, predicting pathological stage and prognosis following treatments, based on pre-operative or postoperative variables, that may be used regardless of race [17-19].

Concern that immediate radical treatment may not be necessary for all men with PSA-detected prostate cancer is stimulating ongoing interest in conservative approaches [20-22] **(Ib/A)**. Published radical prostatectomy series suggest that 20%-30% of men have pathologically insignificant cancer at the time of diagnosis, based on volume and grade [23,24]. Epidemiological and screening studies also raise concern about the consequence of over-diagnosis [25,26]. At the Johns Hopkins Hospital, USA, clinical and pathological criteria have been identified to select and monitor (older) men with localised prostate cancer who may be managed expectantly [27]. These criteria include PSA density less than 0.15ng/ml/cc and favourable biopsy findings. Favourable biopsy findings are indicated by a Gleason score of less than 7, fewer than three cores involved and less than 50% involvement in any core. Biopsy Gleason pattern 4 or 5, two cores with more than 50% cancer and a PSA density greater than 0.15, have been shown to predict more extensive disease. These criteria have been shown to be clinically useful in older selected patients, and biomarkers may contribute in future to prediction of biologically significant disease.

This man has severe symptoms, poor uroflow and large residual volume at a relatively young age, and further evaluation would be prudent prior to any definitive decision. Treatment strategy will be focused on cancer control, and for each therapeutic option, potential benefit must be considered alongside the profile of complications, potential morbidity and effects on quality of life. In addition, for each option, the significance and management of pre-existing lower urinary tract symptoms must also be taken into consideration in the cancer treatment strategy. In relieving prostatic outflow obstruction, radical prostatectomy may reduce urinary symptoms and thereby substantially benefit quality of life [28,29]. The possibility and potential significance of other urodynamic abnormalities, such as detrusor hypocontractility, also warrant consideration, and detrusor instability, in particular, may be associated with postoperative difficulty with urinary control: such diagnoses must however, be considered within a wider setting of clinical and objective assessment [30]. Routine cystoscopy prior to radical prostatectomy may be worthwhile in individual cases, particularly to

exclude concomitant pathologies, but overall, it has a low diagnostic yield [31,32]. Where lower urinary tract symptoms and signs are secondary to prostatic outflow obstruction, improvement in uroflow, bladder emptying and quality of life may be anticipated [33].

Interstitial brachytherapy: Case 1

Interstitial brachytherapy (IB) would be an excellent treatment for the cancer described in this vignette. Single-institution, retrospective reports indicate that favourable risk cancers (PSA <10, Gleason <7, T1-2) are cured in most cases with IB alone [1,2] **(II/B)**. No prospective, multi-institutional trials on the long-term efficacy of IB have been published. The Radiation Therapy Oncology Group has completed accrual to two single arm phase II studies that seek to determine the GI and GU morbidity of IB alone or combined with external beam radiation therapy in a multi-institutional setting. The American College of Surgeons Oncology Group (ACOSOG) has opened a phase III trial comparing the efficacy of radical prostatectomy and IB.

The characteristics of the patient in whom this cancer resides, however, make IB significantly less appealing. Retrospective reports have examined the relationship between IPSS at diagnosis and urinary morbidity following IB. Men with higher IPSS scores prior to IB experience more acute urinary retention, longer duration of urinary symptoms and are more likely to undergo TURP following IB [3,4] **(II/B)**. High pre-treatment IPSS is an exclusion criterion for at least three prospective, multi-institutional trials of IB (RTOG 98-05, RTOG P-0019, ACOSOG Z0070).

The young age of this gentleman may concern some but there is no strong evidence to suggest that young men fare any better or worse with brachytherapy compared to other options. On the other hand, this patient is expected to live another 25 years (USA Census Estimates, 2001) and would be at risk for late radiation-induced morbidity. The long-term (>20 years) morbidity of IB is not well studied. It is clear from the MGH proton beam trial that GI morbidity tends to occur within five years of treatment but GU morbidity continues to appear for several years following treatment [5] **(II/B)**. In summary, this cancer is likely to be cured with IB but characteristics of the patient persuade this clinician to recommend an alternative strategy such as radical prostatectomy.

External beam radiotherapy: Case 1

This young black man has a T1c moderately differentiated adenocarcinoma of the prostate with a low risk of both seminal vesicle (3.6%) and pelvic lymph node (2.4%) involvement, using the Roach and modified Roach formulae [3]. Radical prostatectomy would allow definitive pathological staging and many patients are upstaged at the time of surgery [1, 2, 4, 5] **(Ia/A)**. In this racial group, there is known to be poorer stage-for-stage outcome [6] **(Ia/A)**; thus, non-surgical treatment may result in understaging. External beam radiotherapy necessitates daily treatment for seven to eight weeks and has been extensively reviewed in early stage disease [7, 8] **(IIa/B)**. Historically, control rates range from 43%-98% (Table 1). Like radical prostatectomy, external beam radiation therapy has

undergone a technological revolution, in particular, the development of conformal radiotherapy, increasing the accuracy with which high-dose radiation beams may be shaped to the target volume, with relative sparing of the surrounding normal tissue and hence, allowing dose escalation [9] **(Ib/A)**. This provides a radiobiological advantage as doses above 64 Gy (previous standard UK dose) have been shown to significantly improve both local control and survival, particularly when serum PSA levels are >10ng/ml [9] **(Ib/A)** (Table 2).

Results from radiation show survival comparable to surgery, but with other side effects. In such a young man, potency and continence are key issues to maintain quality of life.

Potency preservation rates for external beam radiotherapy are higher than for standard non-nerve-sparing prostatectomy [10, 11] **(III/B)** and similar or slightly higher than in unilateral or bilateral nerve-sparing prostatectomy (up to 50%). Post-radiotherapy potency may be sensitive to sildenafil [11,12]. Low-grade

Table 1. Results of conventional radiotherapy.

Study	Patient number	Clinical stage	DFS	CFS
Hanks 1994 [13]	104	T1b-T2	67% 10 year	86% 10 year
Fowler 1995 [26]	138	A2	43% 10 year	86% 10 year
Zietman 1995 [8]	504	T1-T2	65% 10 year	-
Perez 1995 [27]	16	A1	100% 10 year	-
	112	A2	69% 10 year	-
	373	B	57% 10 year	-
Kuban 1995 [28]	27	A2	66% 10 year	83% 10 year
	60	B1	57% 10 year	93% 10 year
	246	B2	48% 10 year	78% 10 year
Hahn 1996 [29]	15	T1a	100% 10 year	-
	135	T1b	98% 10 year	-
	77	T2a	88% 10 year	-
	269	T2b	63% 10 year	-
Pollack 1998 [30]	643	T1-T2	Dose >67 Gy, 87% 4-year freedom from failure Dose <67 Gy, 67% 4-year freedom from failure	-
Horwitz 1998 [31]	568	T1-T2	99% 5-year BFFF	-

DFS=Disease-free survival; CFS=Cause-specific survival; BFFF=Biochemical free from failure using ASTRO consensus of three successive PSA rises.

Table 2. Conformal radiotherapy results.

Study	Patient number	BFFF
Roach [32]	501 T1-T2	
	Initial PSA:	
	<4	90% 4 year
	4-10	60% 4 year
	10-20	35% 4 year
	>20	30% 4 year
Zelefsky 1998 [33]	213 T1-T2**	
	Initial PSA:	
	<10	93% 5 year
	10-20	60% 5 year
	>20	40% 5 year
Pollack 2002 [9]	305 T1-T3	
	Initial PSA:	No dose effect
	<10	75% 6 year
	>10	Dose 78 Gy: 62% 6 year; Dose 70 Gy: 43% 6 year

BFFF=Biochemical free from failure with PSA<1ng/ml; ** received 3 months neoadjuvant hormones pre-radiotherapy

urinary side effects occur frequently during external beam irradiation [10,13] but high-grade toxicity is rare. This man has significant pre-treatment obstructive symptoms and these may worsen after definitive radiation treatment. Acute and late bowel and rectal morbidity are observed with radiotherapy, although these can be reduced with a conformal technique. There is 1%-2% risk of severe rectal bleeding [10] with a 20%-25% risk of varying degrees of long-term bowel dysfunction (IIa/B).

Radiotherapy is a treatment option for this man and we would advise 3D conformal radiotherapy to the prostate with a margin of 1cm to cover any sub-clinical disease and allow for organ motion and changes in daily patient set-up. He would be treated to a dose of 74 Gy in 37 daily fractions over 7½ weeks. However, given his pre-existing severe urinary symptoms, concerns would arise with regard to significant deterioration of urinary function during radiotherapy and in the immediate post-radiation period. A pre-radiation transurethral resection of the prostate may be required and depending on the size of the prostate (not given), he may require neoadjuvant hormone therapy in the form of an LHRH analogue, which in itself would affect potency and general quality of life.

Case 2

This 69-year-old man has had a PSA test and DRE as part of investigation of moderate urinary tract symptoms (IPSS 21). He is not bothered by his established sexual dysfunction. He is found to have clinical stage T2a prostate cancer, a PSA of 6.8ng/ml with bilateral Gleason pattern 4 in up to 40% of four of six cores, and perineural invasion. There is no family history of prostate cancer. TRUS shows the prostate with a volume around 40ml.

Radical prostatectomy: Case 2

Therapeutic decisions must integrate clinical assessment of prostate cancer in relation to life expectancy, comorbidity and the wishes of an informed individual. This case raises difficult issues of case selection as it relates to patient age and pathological assessment of the tumour. If this 69-year-old man did not have prostate cancer, and was fit and well, without significant comorbidities, he would have a life expectancy of at least ten years. Radical prostatectomy is routinely carried out in men in their seventh decade, and indeed, older. However, survival benefit is less likely with advancing age, owing to limited life expectancy and death from other causes [34,35] **(Ib/A)**.

The need for curative treatment of prostate cancer and its benefit strongly relate to age and comorbidity, as well as the tumour itself [36]. Unfortunately, for any individual patient, neither life expectancy nor the absolute benefit of various alternative interventions, present or future, can be predicted reliably. Age becomes a more critical factor as it increases, not least because assumptions invoked in making recommendations become less certain. In the very elderly, of course, concurrent illness and limited life expectancy become of more immediate significance. Adoption of rigid guidelines recommending specific treatments in relation to age can therefore be extremely difficult. Further issues related to patient age are discussed in Case 4, a man of 72 years. It is relevant to observe that in the USA, radical prostatectomy rates in older men have declined in recent years [37].

Recommendations for treatment will focus on reduction in risk of future metastasis. Tumours of this grade, managed expectantly, have a strong tendency to progress to metastatic disease over a ten-year period, which is within this individual's life expectancy [5,6]. If the tumour is truly localised, radical prostatectomy may be curative. However, the risk of undetectable micrometastatic disease may not be insignificant, eventually manifesting with subsequent biochemical recurrence and progression [38]. The risk and time to metastatic progression relate to tumour grade, time to biochemical recurrence and PSA doubling time. A potential benefit of radical prostatectomy in controlling local disease in patients developing distant progression is not prospectively defined. For higher-grade tumours, PSA control or low PSA doubling time, following radical definitive treatment, can be associated with excellent long-term metastases-free survival. It may be conjectured that such outcomes may not be so reliably achieved by treatment leaving the prostate with high-risk disease *in situ*.

The biopsy findings indicate that this man has a significant risk of extraprostatic disease [39] **(IIa/B)**. Based on clinical stage, serum PSA, and biopsy

Gleason score, Partin's table predicts a probability of organ-confined cancer of 33%, 52% risk of established capsular penetration and 10% risk of seminal vesicle involvement. The presence of Gleason pattern 4 bilaterally, in four of six cores and the presence of biopsy perineural invasion also indicate a significant risk of adverse pathological findings [40-42]. As discussed previously, his advanced age may also be associated with more advanced pathological stage disease. In such circumstances, meticulous surgical technique may contribute to minimising the risk of positive surgical margins [43,44] **(IIa/B)**. Considerations pertaining to pathological stage and surgical margin status relate to the risk of established micrometastatic disease and recurrent or progressive disease following local therapy [4].

In carefully selected patients with high-grade localised prostate cancer, radical prostatectomy nevertheless may be appropriate and achieve disease control [45] **(IIa/B)**. Although neoadjuvant hormone therapy has been shown to downstage the local pathological stage, no reduction in risk of subsequent disease progression has been observed [46]. The risk that radical prostatectomy alone will not control this man's disease relates to pathological findings that can only be established after operation [39]. Factors that determine any long-term benefit from subsequent (adjuvant) radiation [47], and the optimal timing of later hormone intervention are important in this context [48,49]. Both impose additional side effects, and at present, rely on considerations of disease "risk" or biochemical recurrence [50,51]. For an individual with such extensive high-grade disease, radical prostatectomy cannot assure metastatic control, and the side effects may additionally and adversely affect quality of life.

In the presence of established metastases, radical prostatectomy has a limited role in prostate cancer treatment **(IIa/B)**. Where the risk of metastatic disease cannot be considered minimal, additional information may be appropriate prior to further therapeutic considerations. Particularly in "high risk" cases, magnetic resonance imaging (MRI), and to a lesser extent, computerised tomography (CT), have been used to define local extent of disease and regional lymph node status. Prostascint scanning, particularly in combination with CT, may also be useful